Case Reports in Pediatric Dentistry

Edited by
Evert van Amerongen
Maddelon de Jong-Lenters
Luc Marks
Jaap Veerkamp

Case Reports in Pediatric Dentistry

Edited by
Evert van Amerongen
Maddelon de Jong-Lenters
Luc Marks
Jaap Veerkamp

QUINTESSENCE PUBLISHING

Quintessence Publishing Co Ltd
London, Berlin, Chicago, Tokyo, Barcelona, Beijing, Istanbul, Milan,
Moscow, New Delhi, Paris, Prague, São Paulo, Seoul and Warsaw

Quintessence

British Library Cataloguing in Publication Data

Case reports in pediatric dentistry.
1. Pedodontics--Case studies.
I. Amerongen, Evert van.
617.6'45-dc22

ISBN-13: 9781850971962

QUINTESSENCE PUBLISHING

Quintessence Publishing Co. Ltd,
Grafton Road, New Malden, Surrey KT3 3AB,
Great Britain
www.quintpub.co.uk

Editing: Quintessence Publishing Co. Ltd, London
Layout and Production: Jens Girke, Quintessenz Verlags-GmbH, Berlin
Printing and binding: Mercedes-Druck, Berlin
Printed in Germany

Foreword

It is essential that clinicians treating children have a high degree of awareness and knowledge of a wide range of oral conditions to optimize the dental care for their patients. Some of these conditions are commonly encountered whereas others are rather infrequent, thus giving the practicing dentist limited experience to build up diagnostic and treatment skills. The latter may concern, for example, different types of developmental disturbances such as hypodontia or disturbances of mineralization of dental hard tissues, as well as pathologic conditions in oral mucosa and bone. Of great interest in increasing knowledge and clinical experiences is the case reports/presentations, which, unfortunately to a limited extent, are published in pediatric scientific journals. This book has been produced in an attempt to overcome this and to give dentists involved in clinical dentistry for children an opportunity to a systematic approach in continuing education in diagnostics, indications, treatment, and follow-up of cases that could be seen in their own practices.

In this book, 16 cases treated by experienced clinicians are presented, including case history, examination, diagnosis, indications for treatment, treatment options, and evaluation/prognosis. References for further reading are also given. The clinical pictures and radiographs are of excellent quality. The ambition of the editors to present a new book with new cases every other year is to be commended. This means that we can expect a library of first-class case presentations, which over time will be of great importance for high quality care in dentistry for children.

The present book is an outstanding, important contribution to achieving high standards in clinical children's dentistry and also to stimulate discussions on treatment strategies. The book should be available to all clinicians involved in dental care for children, it should be used in education, and to form a "case library" in all clinics/practices. This book can therefore be highly recommended.

Göran Koch

Preface

In the Netherlands, as in several other countries in Europe and other parts of the world, there are specialist training programs in pediatric dentistry. Postgraduate students are expected to collect many case reports during this program. They get the opportunity to present these cases to only a limited number of colleagues, and after completion of their training there is a considerable chance that those case reports disappear in a drawer. This observation was the basis of the idea to publish a series of books on those case reports in the Netherlands to give our Dutch colleagues the opportunity to learn from all these cases. However, after the publication of the first two volumes, it appeared that there was also a need and interest in neighboring countries for such purely clinically oriented books on pediatric dentistry. This interest set us the challenge to produce an identical book in English, with case reports from different countries.

This book is unique in pediatric dentistry; although there are many textbooks on children's dentistry, there was a need for a concise collection of case reports. I hope that this book will not only serve as a reference for specialists in pediatric dentistry, but also help general practitioners in solving clinical problems related to their pediatric patients.

On behalf of the authors,

Evert van Amerongen

Editors

Dr W Evert van Amerongen, *Head of the Section of Pedodontology, Department of Cariology Endodontology Pedodontology and Oral Microbiology, Academic Centre for Dentistry in Amsterdam (ACTA), Amsterdam, The Netherlands*

Dr Maddelon de Jong-Lenters, *Pediatric Dentist, Pediatric Dental Practice Cleyburch Noordwijk; Special Dental Care Centre MCA (Medical Centre Alkmaar) and Cariology Endodontology Pedodontology and Oral Microbiology, Academic Centre for Dentistry in Amsterdam (ACTA), Amsterdam, The Netherlands*

Prof. Dr Luc Marks, *Pediatric Dentist, Pediatric Dental Department and Centre of Special Dental Care, University of Gent, Gent, Belgium*

Dr Jaap SJ Veerkamp, *Pediatric Dentist, Department of Cariology Endodontology Pedodontology and Oral Microbiology, Academic Centre for Dentistry in Amsterdam (ACTA), Amsterdam, The Netherlands*

Authors

Satu Alaluusua
Department of Paediatric and Preventive Dentistry, Institute of Dentistry, University of Helsinki, Finland, and Department of Oral and Maxillofacial Diseases and Hospital for Children and Adolescents, Helsinki University Central Hospital, Helsinki, Finland

Heikki Alapulli
Department of Oral and Maxillofacial Diseases and Hospital for Children and Adolescents, Helsinki University Central Hospital, Helsinki, Finland

Veslemøy E. Bjørkeng
Pediatric Dentist, Risvollan Public Dental Clinic, Trondheim, Norway

Katharina Bücher
Department of Conservative Dentistry and Periodontology, Ludwig Maximilian University of Munich, Germany

Roeland De Moor
Department of Operative Dentistry and Endodontology, Ghent Dental Laser Centre, Dental School, Ghent University Hospital, Ghent University, Belgium

Monty Duggal
Dental Institute, Department of Paediatric Dentistry, Leeds, UK

Ivar Espelid
Department of Paediatric Dentistry and Behavioural Science, Faculty of Dentistry, University of Oslo, Norway

Dafydd Evans
Senior Lecturer, Preventive and Children's Section, Dundee Dental Hospital and School, Dundee, Scotland

Mario Fazzi
Dentistry Unit, Department of Head and Neck, University of Parma, Italy

Roland Frankenberger
Dental Clinic 1 – Operative Dentistry and Periodontology, University Medical Center, Erlangen, Germany

Reinhard Hickel
Department of Conservative Dentistry and Periodontology, Ludwig Maximilian University of Munich, Germany

Marie Therese Hosey
Department of Paediatric Dentistry, King's College London Dental Institute, London, UK

Marie-Charlotte Huysmans
Division of Preventive and Curative Care, College of Dentistry, Radboud University Medical Centre, Radboud University Nijmegen, The Netherlands

Nicola Innes
Clinical Lecturer, Preventive and Children's Section, Dundee Dental Hospital and School, Dundee, Scotland

Norbert Krämer
Department of Paediatric Dentistry, University Medical Center Carl Gustv Carus, Dresden, Germany

Jan Kühnisch
Department of Conservative Dentistry and Periodontology, Ludwig Maximilian University of Munich, Germany

Manfredi Maddalena
Dentistry Unit, Department of Head and Neck, University of Parma, Italy

Marie-Cècile Manière
Department of Paediatric Dentistry, Louis Pasteur University, Strasbourg, France

Luc C. Martens
Department of Paediatric Dentistry and Special Care, Ghent University, Belgium

Rèmy Mathis
Department of Orthodontics, Louis Pasteur University, Strasbourg, France

Julie Caroline Mitchell
Department of Paediatric Dentistry, King's College London Dental Institute, London, UK

Anne Grethe Myhre
Paediatric Department, Rikshospitalet University Hospital, Oslo, Norway

Frèdèric Obry
Department of Paediatric Dentistry, Louis Pasteur University, Strasbourg, France

Marleen Peumans
Department of Conservative Dentistry, School of Dentistry, Oral Pathology and Maxillo-Facial Surgery, Catholic University of Leuven, Belgium

Silvia Pizzi
Dentistry Unit, Department of Head and Neck, University of Parma, Italy

Andrea Savi
Dentistry Unit, Department of Head and Neck, University of Parma, Italy

Sven Simonsen
Paediatric Department, Sykehuset Østfold, Norway

Anne B. Skaare
Department of Paediatric Dentistry and Behavioural Science, Faculty of Dentistry, University of Oslo, Norway

Ilija Skrinjaric
Department of Paediatric Dentistry, School of Dental Medicine, University of Zagreb, Croatia

Gert Stel
Division of Preventive and Curative Care, College of Dentistry, Radboud University Medical Centre, Radboud University Nijmegen, The Netherlands

Anna Lena Sundell
Department of Paediatric Dentistry, Institute for Postgraduate Dental Education, Jönköping, Sweden

Marco Tamani
Dentistry Unit, Department of Head and Neck, University of Parma, Italy

Table of Contents

1

Long-term Management of Early Childhood Caries

Norbert Krämer
Roland Frankenberger

Key words: early childhood caries, nursing bottle caries, adhesive restoration, dentures

Age category: 0–4 and 4–7 years

Definition

Early childhood caries (ECC) is "the occurrence of any sign of dental caries on any tooth surface (non-cavitated or cavitated lesions) during the first 3 years of life".[1] Severe early childhood caries (S-ECC) is present when children younger than 3 years show any sign of smooth-surface caries. At the age >5 years, S-ECC is present when one or more cavitated, missing (due to caries), or filled smooth surfaces are found in primary maxillary anterior teeth or when there is a DMF score of ≥4 (age 3, Figs 1-1a, 1-1b), ≥5 (age 4, Fig. 1-2), or ≥6 (age 5).[2] The so-called "nursing caries" (NC) is a special kind of ECC, in which decay is localized to the maxillary anterior primary teeth. NC is diagnosed when two or more labial or palatal surfaces of the maxillary primary incisors show carious lesions (Figs 1-3a,1-3b).

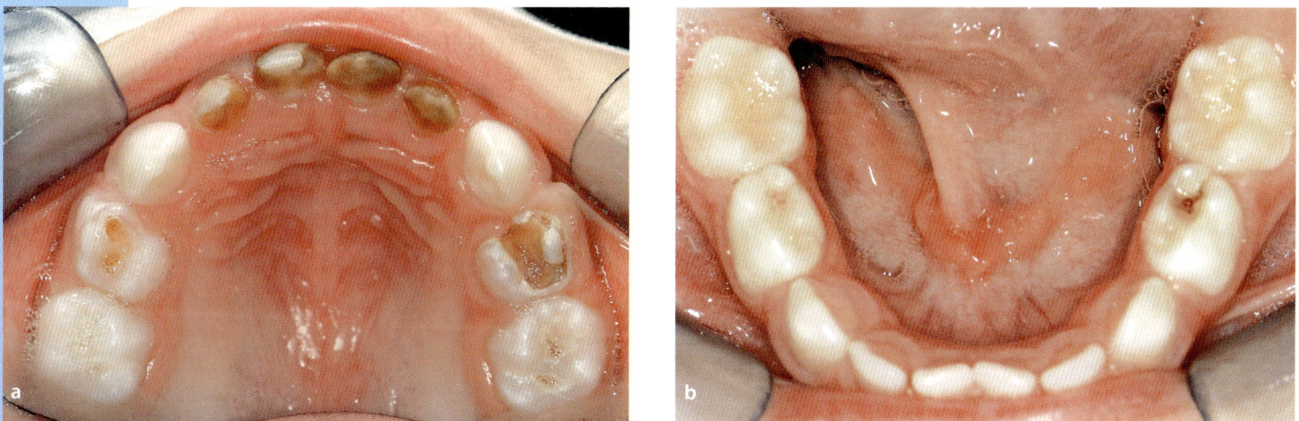

a b

Fig. 1-1a,b A 3-year old boy with typical early childhood caries (ECC). He was given a nursing bottle at night for the first 2 years of his life. Although the practice was stopped, the disease progressed. 1-1a The occlusal lesions in the maxillary right and left primary second molars (55, 65) demonstrate the treatment need. 1-1b Occlusal lesions in the mandibular left and right primary first molars (74, 84). Altogether, 10 teeth are decayed.

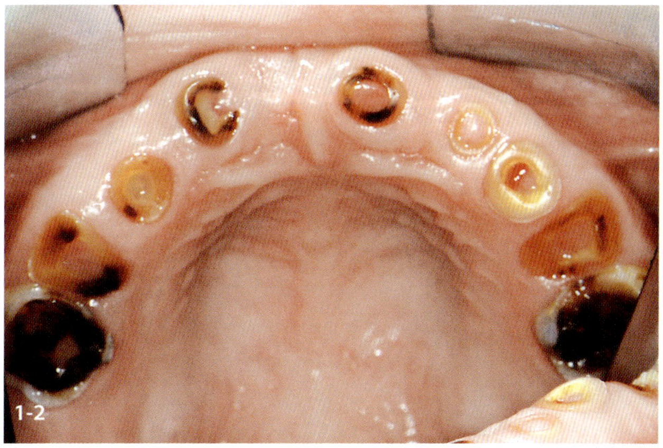

1-2

Fig. 1-2 A 4.5-year old girl with completely destroyed maxillary primary teeth. On the basis of the age of the patient and the considerable number of decayed teeth, severe early childhood caries was diagnosed.

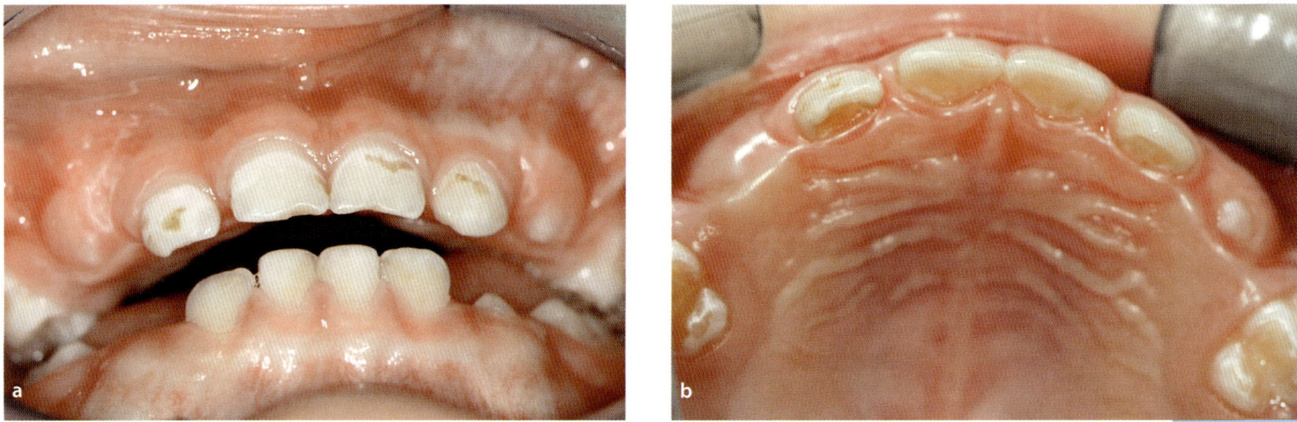

Fig. 1-3a Typical appearance of nursing caries in a 22-month boy. Even at this age, the labial surfaces exhibit signs of severe early childhood caries.

Fig. 1-3b Palatal view of the patient in Figure 1-3a: the maxillary right primary lateral incisor (52) has a progressive lesion. The reason for the decay was nightly use of baby bottles with fruit juice.

Data on risk factors for ECC are not consistently reported. In developed countries, the main reasons are nightly use of nursing bottles with sweet drinks, poor parental understanding of oral hygiene, prolonged contact of the teeth with sweet drinks, lower socioeconomic status, and ethnic background.[3] Some authors have described a more complex etiology, ie, the degree of interaction among the factors: infection with mutans streptococci, social status, family structure and social networks, and use of baby bottles or nursing on demand.[4]

Possibilities and limits of restorative treatment of the decayed primary dentition are determined by: time of intervention, degree of decay, compliance of the child, and the preventive behaviors of the parents and children.

THE PROBLEM

Maggie visited us for the first time at 2.7 years of age, with severe decay of her maxillary anterior teeth (Fig. 1-4). She did not have any pain. The central incisors had fractured 2 weeks before, which is when her mother realized that her teeth had brownish discoloration. Maggie's mother should have been educated about early childhood caries, because her 10 years older sister also had ECC and had been treated under general anesthesia (GA) several years before. Because of this, the mother desired similar treatment for Maggie.

CASE DESCRIPTION

History

Maggie was diagnosed as having Mohr syndrome (oro-facial-digital syndrome type II) shortly after birth. Due to the presence of typical features of this syndrome (hypoplasia of the body of the mandible; bilateral polysyndactyly; conductive hearing defect; wide root of the nose and telecanthus [ie, increased distance between the medial eye angles]), she was under long-term medical care. When she came to the dental clinic for the first time, her redundant toes had already been removed, and the operative removal of her redundant fingers had been planned. There was no history of this autosomal-recessive disease on the maternal side of the family. The patient's development appeared retarded for her age and communication was impossible. She had not received any dental care before because the mother did not have confidence in the local dentists. Therefore, she had now brought Maggie to the university clinic.

Maggie's oral hygiene was moderate, although the mother was motivated. Owing to resistance by the daughter, additional brushing by the mother was only possible as a forced action. According

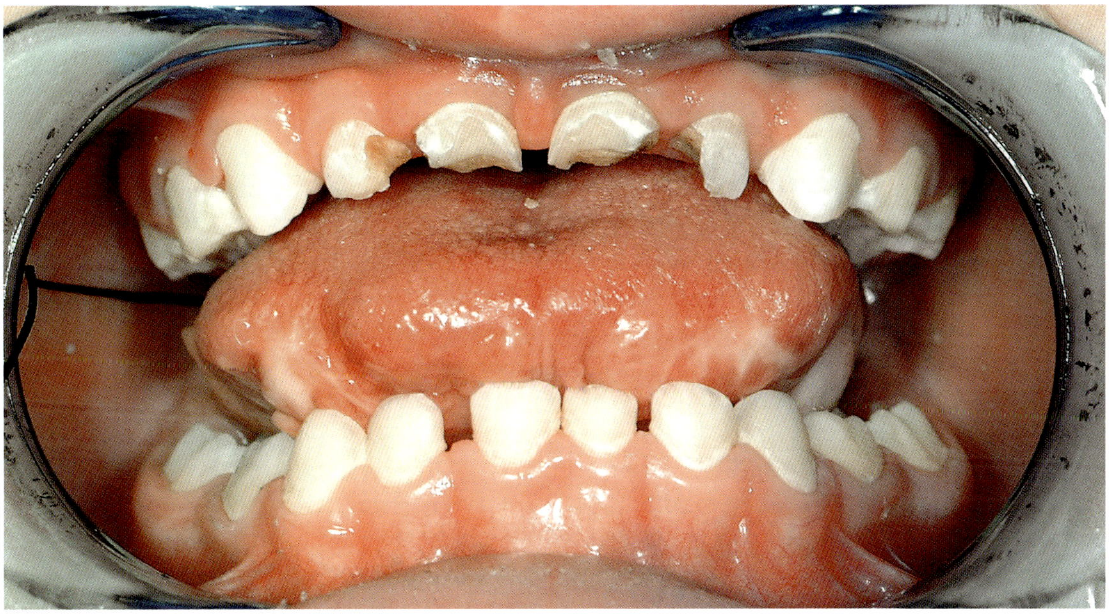

Fig. 1-4 Initial findings. Due to poor compliance, these findings were recorded under general anesthesia. The mesiobuccal aspect of the maxillary right primary first molar (54) shows initial decay. All other teeth except for the maxillary anterior teeth were sound.

to the mother, the patient's teeth were brushed twice daily with fluoride-containing (500 ppm) children's toothpaste. Fluoride tablets were discontinued after her second birthday. Food history showed that after breastfeeding was stopped, between 6 and 12 months of age, she had a baby bottle with thinned fruit juice or milk throughout the day and at night.

Maggie had three older half-siblings from her mother's first marriage. The mother had separated from her father a year ago and was now a single mother, caring for her children (aged 3–16) all alone.

Examination

The maxillary primary incisors (52, 51, 61, 62) showed deep dentinal lesions, but the pulp was not exposed. The palatal decay had progressed to the gingival level (Fig. 1-4). On the mesiobuccal aspect of the maxillary right primary first molar (54), a white-opaque initial carious lesion was detected without probing. No swelling or fistula was detected.

Additional Investigations

All attempts to take radiographs failed.

DIAGNOSIS

On the basis of the patient's age and the number and distribution of carious lesions in the primary teeth, S-ECC was diagnosed. The presence of risk factors and localization of the decay primarily to the anterior teeth led to the further diagnosis of NC.

TREATMENT OPTIONS

Definitive

- Extraction of the anterior teeth under GA and replacement with a children's denture.

Alternatives

- Pulpectomy of the four maxillary primary incisors with adhesive restorations.
- Crowns for the maxillary incisors.

Rationale

Adhesive restorations of primary incisors are indicated when the degree of decay allows adequate moisture control, ie, the caries should not extend below the gingiva. Waggoner[5] reported adhesive anterior restorations to be successful in 50–100% of cases. Restorations in teeth that have undergone pulpectomy with iodoform pastes are more likely to fail.[6] Also, use of prefabricated and veneered steel crowns is limited due to high risk of failure. Main reasons for failure are chipping of the white esthetic facing, fracture, or wear.[5]

In the present case, the treatment was carried out under GA because of the poor compliance of the child. Eidelman et al.[7] demonstrated a significantly better treatment outcome under GA compared with the use of conscious sedation. For our patient, it was unclear at that point whether her compliance would increase with time, making further ambulant treatments possible. Also, the requirement for radiographic documentation after pulpectomy could not be fulfilled without GA.[8] So considering all factors, extractions seemed to be the right decision.

A denture was indicated due to the general condition of the patient, with central facial hypoplasia and delayed speech development. Moreover, the patient had started to attend kindergarten and she may have been at a disadvantage in the absence of replacements for her incisors. This situation may have led to difficulty in speech, decreased masticatory efficiency, development of abnormal tongue habits and subsequent malocclusion, and psychological problems.

The aim of treatment with removable denture prosthesis is the re-establishment of esthetics, phonetics, and function while assuring at the same time a high standard of oral hygiene. The continuing growth of the jaws and the changes in the dentition of a child must be closely monitored. Moreover, there should always be enough compliance to take the impression without GA.

> ***Key Message***
> *Any uncertain restoration of primary teeth involves the danger of repeated treatments. For patients of very young age, this also means repeated use of GA.*

TREATMENT AND FOLLOW-UP

Treatment

One month after the first visit, the mother and child received oral hygiene training, diet advice, and fluoride use instructions. The mother was instructed to discontinue bottle feeding. The primary teeth were coated with sodium fluoride varnish (Fluoridin, Voco, Germany).[9] Another month later, the decayed teeth were extracted under GA. The wounds healed without problems (Fig. 1-5). Two months after the procedure, alginate impressions were taken of both jaws to construct a removable partial denture for replacement of the maxillary incisors (52–62). The protruded and elongated mandibular incisors complicated the positioning of the denture teeth (Bambino Tooth, Major Industries). The denture was retained with Adam clasps at the maxillary right and left primary second molars (55, 65), and with C clasps on the maxillary right and left primary canines (53, 63). No screw was incorporated in the denture (Fig. 1-6).

Posttreatment Evaluation 1/Follow-up 1

Maggie visited our office at 3-month intervals. Besides a checkup of the denture, professional tooth cleaning was carried out (polish with brush and paste) and fluoride varnish applied to help her get used to the dental clinic. According to the mother, she had discontinued use of her baby bottles. However, the mother changed her job during that time, and Maggie was predominantly being cared for in the kindergarten and by her older siblings. Therefore, optimal diet control was not possible.

Caries progression became clearly evident (maxillary right primary second molar [55], maxillary right primary first molar [54], maxillary left primary canine [63], maxillary left primary second molar [65], mandibular left primary first molar [74], mandibular right primary canine [83]) 1½ years later. A panoramic radiograph confirmed the clinical findings (Fig. 1-7).

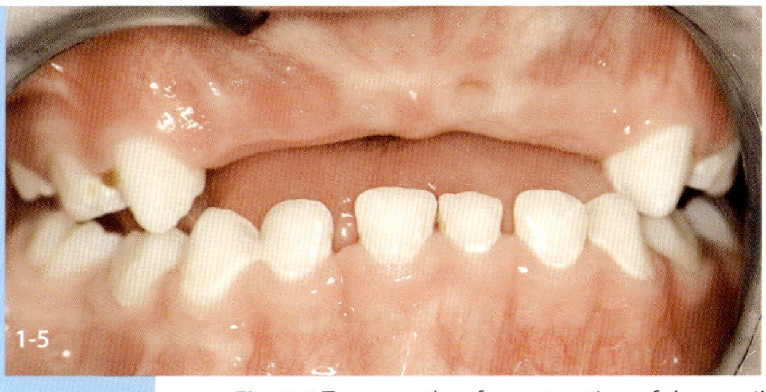

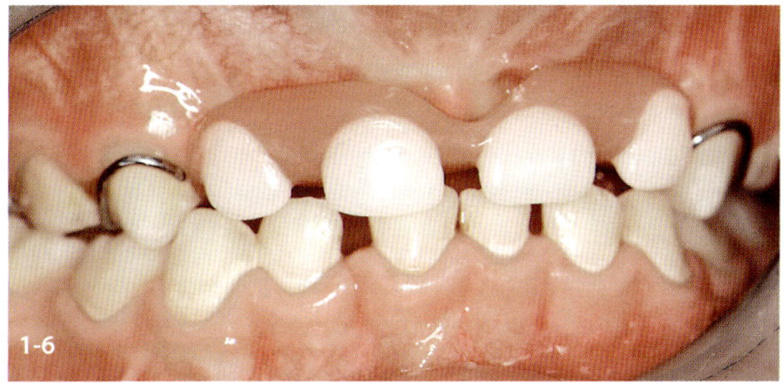

Fig. 1-5 Two months after extraction of the maxillary incisors. The gingival tissues are healthy.

Fig. 1-6 Anterior view of the removable partial denture with integral diastemata. Due to the protrusion and elongation of the mandibular incisors, the maxillary incisors are in a forward position.

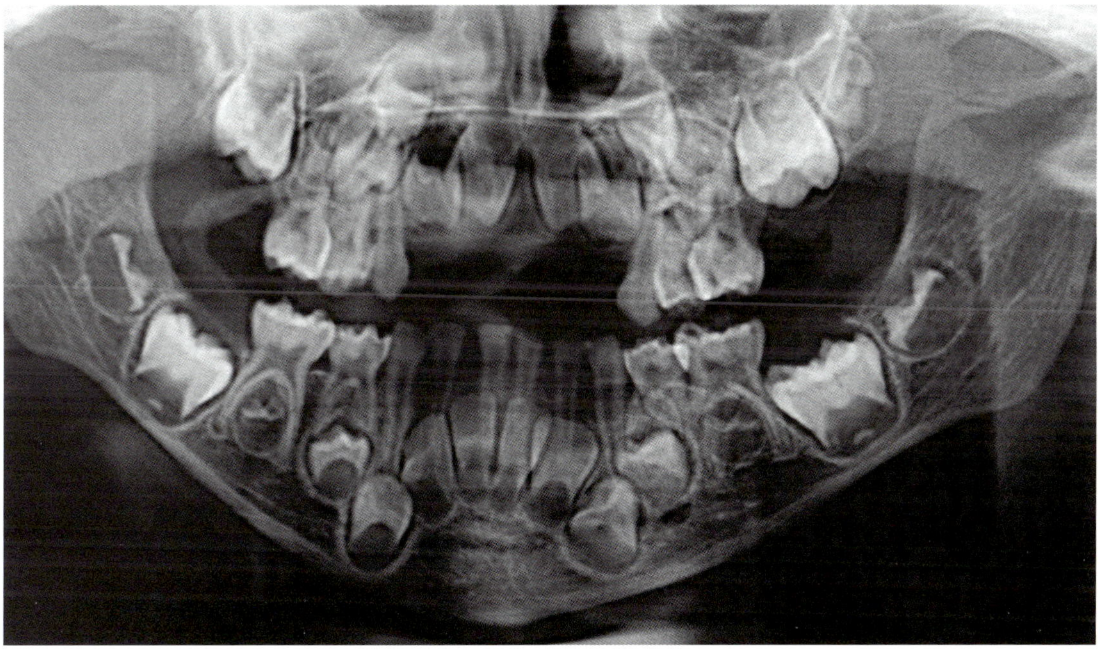

Fig. 1-7 Panoramic radiograph (November 2003). The clinical diagnosis of carious lesions on the mesial aspect of the maxillary right primary first molar (54) and distal aspect of the mandibular left primary first molar (74) was confirmed. Additionally, the mandibular right primary first molar (84) had a distal radiolucency.

FURTHER TREATMENT

Definitive

- Adhesive restorative therapy with bonded compomers and behavioral management.

Alternatives

- Glass-ionomer restorations.
- Resin composites and restorations (with acid-etch technique).
- Prefabricated stainless steel crowns.

Rationale

For restorative therapy, a variety of materials are available on the market. Glass-ionomer cements (GICs) are associated with easy handling and high fluoride release. This makes them especially attractive for Class 1 cavities in uncooperative children. However, their low flexural strength has led to high fracture rates in Class 2 cavities. Further developments (viscous and resin-modified GICs) have improved handling characteristics, but conventional non-resin-modified GICs are still prone to fracture. Compomers exhibit a clear potential as an alternative to amalgam. Long-term results are good even in stress-bearing areas. However, the compliance of the child should last long enough for adhesive application.

Resin composites are still the most time-consuming alternative. When a correct application protocol is followed, resin composites behave in a similar manner to compomers. Therefore, their use has to be considered on a case by case basis. Finally, especially in severely decayed teeth and after endodontic treatment, preformed metal steel crowns should be considered as a last and appropriate alternative to direct restorations.[10] In the present case, due to the esthetic appearance and problems associated with use of nickel, the mother refused crowns. In view of our patient's limited compliance, especially regarding air-water spray, the treatment should have been carried out in small steps and dry conditions. The lesions were too small for being restored with crowns.

Posttreatment Evaluation 2/Follow-up 2

During the following 2 years, new carious lesions (Figs 1-8a, 1-8b) were treated despite persistently poor patient compliance. Figure 1-9 shows the completed treatment. The patient came regularly for prophylactic care with fluoride varnish. During that period, only one proximal lesion in the mandibular right primary first molar (84) required treatment, and a fractured restoration in the mandibular left primary first molar (74) was replaced. Furthermore, the partial denture was monitored. At the age of 6½ years, the permanent maxillary incisors erupted and consequently the labial denture base had to be reduced. Three months later the denture was discontinued (Fig. 1-10).

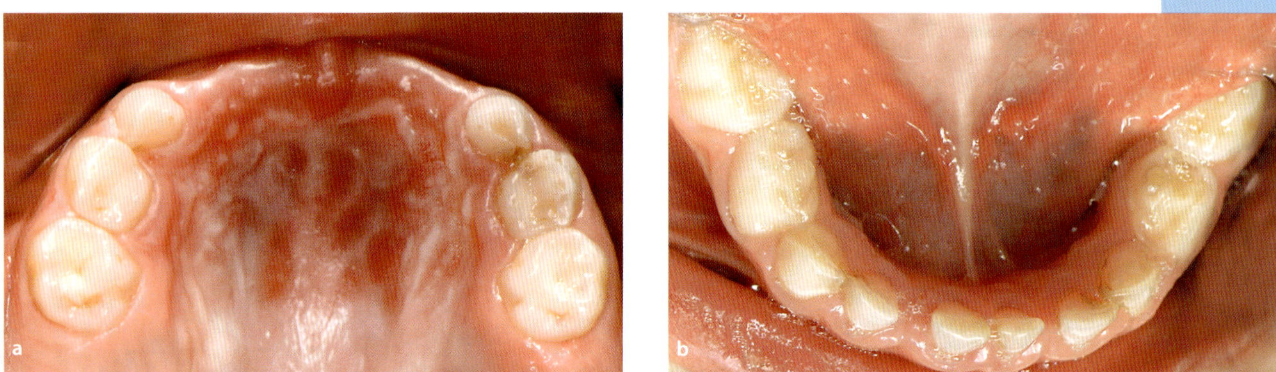

Fig. 1-8a Intraoral view with carious maxillary left primary canine (63) and first molar (64). The palatal restoration in the maxillary right primary second molar (55) is intact, with some staining at the edge of the palatal fissure. The gingiva is altered in the area of the denture base.

Fig. 1-8b Corresponding situation in the mandible. An occlusal glass-ionomer restoration in the mandibular left primary first molar (74) is still intact. Although the surface is moist, the proximal lesion is visible.

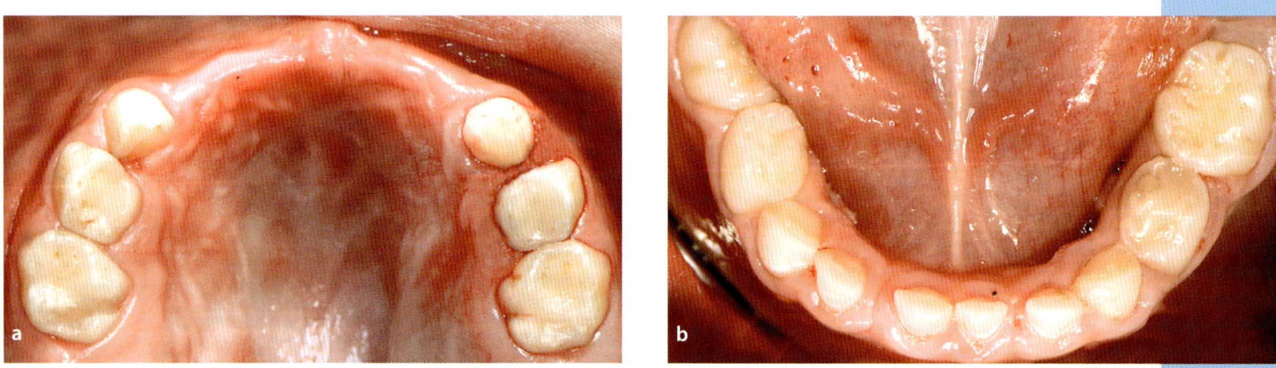

Fig. 1-9a Restoration of the maxillary right primary second molar (55), maxillary left primary canine (63), and the maxillary left primary first and second molars (64, 65) with bonded compomer. To facilitate retention of the removable partial denture, the proximal contact between the maxillary left primary canine (63) and first molar (64) was left open.

Fig. 1-9b Restoration of the mandibular left primary incisors, canine and first molar (71, 72, 73, 74) and the right primary lateral incisor and canine (82, 83). The occlusal GIC filling in the mandibular left first primary molar (74) was not replaced.

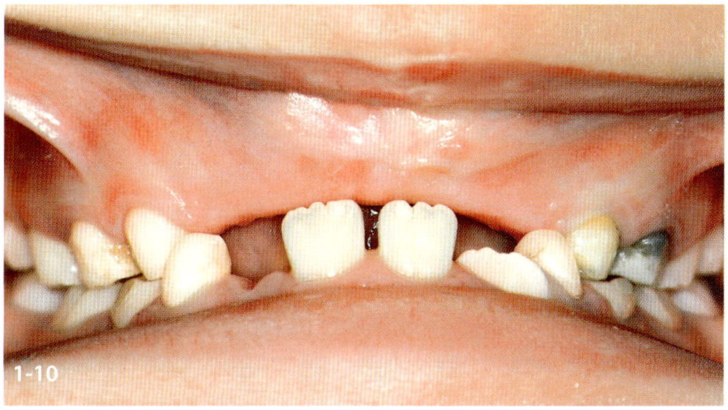

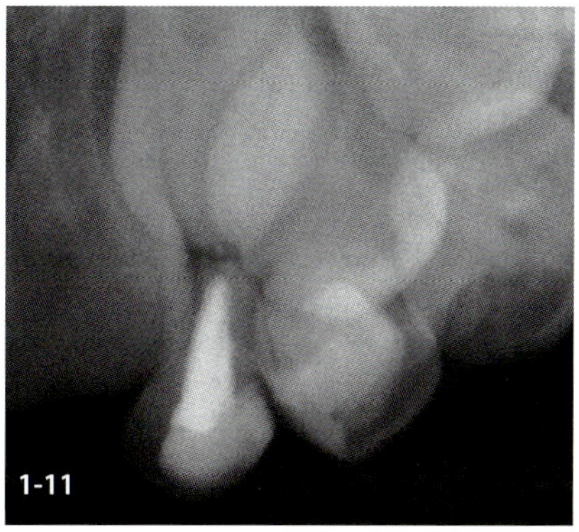

Fig. 1-10 Anterior intraoral view after discontinuation of the partial denture. Due to the hypoplasia of the central face, the lower incisors appear elongated. The maxillary left primary canine and first molar (63, 64) exhibit intrinsic staining following endodontic treatment.

Fig. 1-11 Radiographic appearance of the maxillary left primary canine and first molar (63, 64), 2 years after treatment. No pathology is seen.

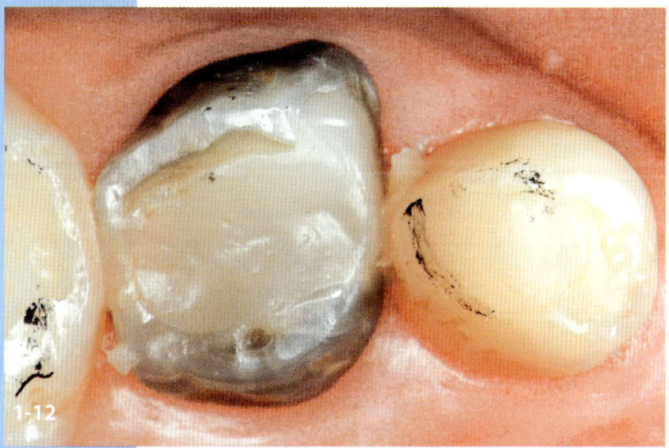

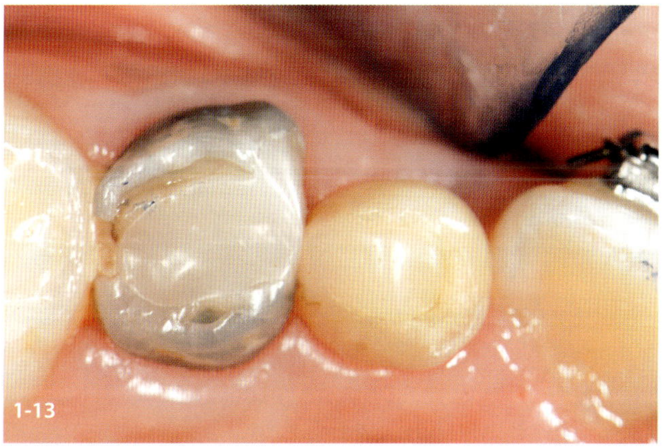

Fig. 1-12 Clinical examination 2 years after treatment under general anesthesia. There is plaque accumulation between the maxillary left primary canine and first molar (63, 64) as well as the two molars (64, 65).

Fig. 1-13 Final recall 3 years after restorative treatment (October 2007). There is a new proximal lesion on the distal aspect of the maxillary left first molar (64); however, the tooth was nearing its time for natural exfoliation.

The patient was referred to an orthodontist, who started treatment for her skeletal problems. Orthodontic treatment is still under way to adjust the overbite by intrusion of the lower incisors, to maximize maxillary development, and to harmonize the jaw relationship.

The radiographic follow-up of the endodontically treated teeth revealed no pathologic changes (Fig. 1-11). The restorations were intact. The maxillary left primary first molar (64) had a grayish stain (Fig. 1-12). Owing to persisting poor oral hygiene, 1 year later the lateral ridge of this tooth was fractured because of proximal caries (Fig. 1-13).

DISCUSSION

Preventive care of S-ECC patients is a considerable challenge for the whole dental and medical team. The present case shows that even after removal of the primary problem (baby bottle), other key risk factors for ECC (socioeconomic status, feeding and weaning history, food habits, oral hygiene, single-parent household) determined the further progress of the disease.[3,11] Therefore, it was important at the beginning of the treatment to extract the teeth with questionable prognosis. Although this was done successfully, including the placement of a partial denture (which incidentally promoted the mother's interest in attending recall appointments) the caries progressed throughout the preschool period.

To prevent problems with jaw development, we decided to treat the patient as conservatively as possible in the long term. The premature loss of the maxillary left primary canine (63) in particular would have been a problem here.

Since compliance got slowly better with age, two different restorative concepts could be applied: GICs have the advantage that these restorations can be placed within 2.5 minutes. In Class 1 cavities, this concept was proven to be successful over the whole period of treatment (Fig. 1-9b, mandibular left primary first molar). In Class 2 cavities, however, the inferior flexural strength of GIC led to the need for several replacements.[10] Adhesive treatment was successful; none of the restorations had to be replaced during the 3 years after the second treatment session under GA.[10] New proximal lesions adjacent to pre-existing fillings were always a problem. Therefore, a stainless steel crown would have been an alternative for the restoration of at least tooth 64. We expect that our patient will require intensive oral care over the next few years or even decades due to her social and medical background. At the last recall visit, molar–incisor hypomineralization (MIH) was diagnosed.

CONCLUSION

This case demonstrates clearly that the diagnosis of ECC can be the first step in a long history of decay, requiring extensive restorative treatment. Currently in Europe, this has led to an increase in debate regarding treatment needs of patients with limited compliance. The pediatric dentist should be the first one to recognize that an early diagnosis of the caries process is the first step in such patients, but it is not a guarantee of success.

REFERENCES

1. Ismail AI. Prevention of early childhood caries. Community Dent Oral Epidemiol 1998;26(1 suppl.):49–61.
2. American Academy of Pediatric Dentistry. Definition of early childhood caries (ECC). Pediatr Dent 2006;28(suppl.):13.
3. Tiberia MJ, Milnes AR, Feigal RJ, Morley KR, Richardson DS, Croft WG, et al. Risk factors for early childhood caries in Canadian preschool children seeking care. Pediatr Dent 2007;29:201–208.
4. Weerheijm K, Uyttendaele-Speybrouck B. Euwe H, Groen H. Prolonged demand breast-feeding and nursing caries. Caries Res 1998;32:46–50.
5. Waggoner WF. Anterior crowns for primary anterior teeth: an evidence based assessment of the literature. Eur Arch Paediatr Dent 2006; 7:53–57.
6. Kupietzky A, Waggoner WF, Galea J. The clinical and radiographic success of bonded resin composite strip crowns for primary incisors. Pediatr Dent 2003;25:577–581.
7. Eidelman E, Faibis S, Peretz B. A comparison of restorations for children with early childhood caries treated under general anesthesia or conscious sedation. Pediatr Dent 2000;22:33–37.
8. Rodd HD, Waterhouse PJ, Fuks AB, Fayle SA, Moffat MA. Pulp therapy for primary molars. Int J Paediatr Dent 2006;16(suppl. 1):15–23.
9. American Academy of Pediatric Dentistry. Policy for early childhood caries (ECC): Classifications, consequences and preventive strategies. Pediatr Dent 2006;27:31–3.
10. Krämer N, Lohbauer U, Frankenberger R. Restorative materials in the primary dentition of poli-caries patients. Eur Arch Paediatr Dent 2007; 8:29–35.
11. Schroth RJ, Cheba V. Determining the prevalence and risk factors for early childhood caries in a community dental health clinic. Pediatr Dent 2007;29:387–396.

2

Hypomineralized Molars

Marleen Peumans

Key words: hypomineralized molar, molar–incisor hypomineralization (MIH), enamel hypomineralization, enamel opacity

Age category: 7–12 years

Definition

A hypomineralized molar is a first permanent molar that has distinct creamy white or yellow-brown opacities, usually in the occlusal third of the crown. These teeth undergo posteruptive enamel breakdown. Often a person experiences sensitivity or pain in these teeth, which may occur spontaneously or while eating and/or drinking. The more appropriate term for this condition is molar–incisor hypomineralization (MIH). This term was introduced in 2001 to describe the clinical phenomenon of acquired enamel hypomineralization of systemic origin, affecting one or more permanent molars with or without a similar defect affecting the incisors (Figs 2-1a to 2-1d, Fig. 2-2).[1] The severity of the damage to the enamel of the molars varies between the teeth even within the same dentition. The hypomineralized enamel may break down after eruption.

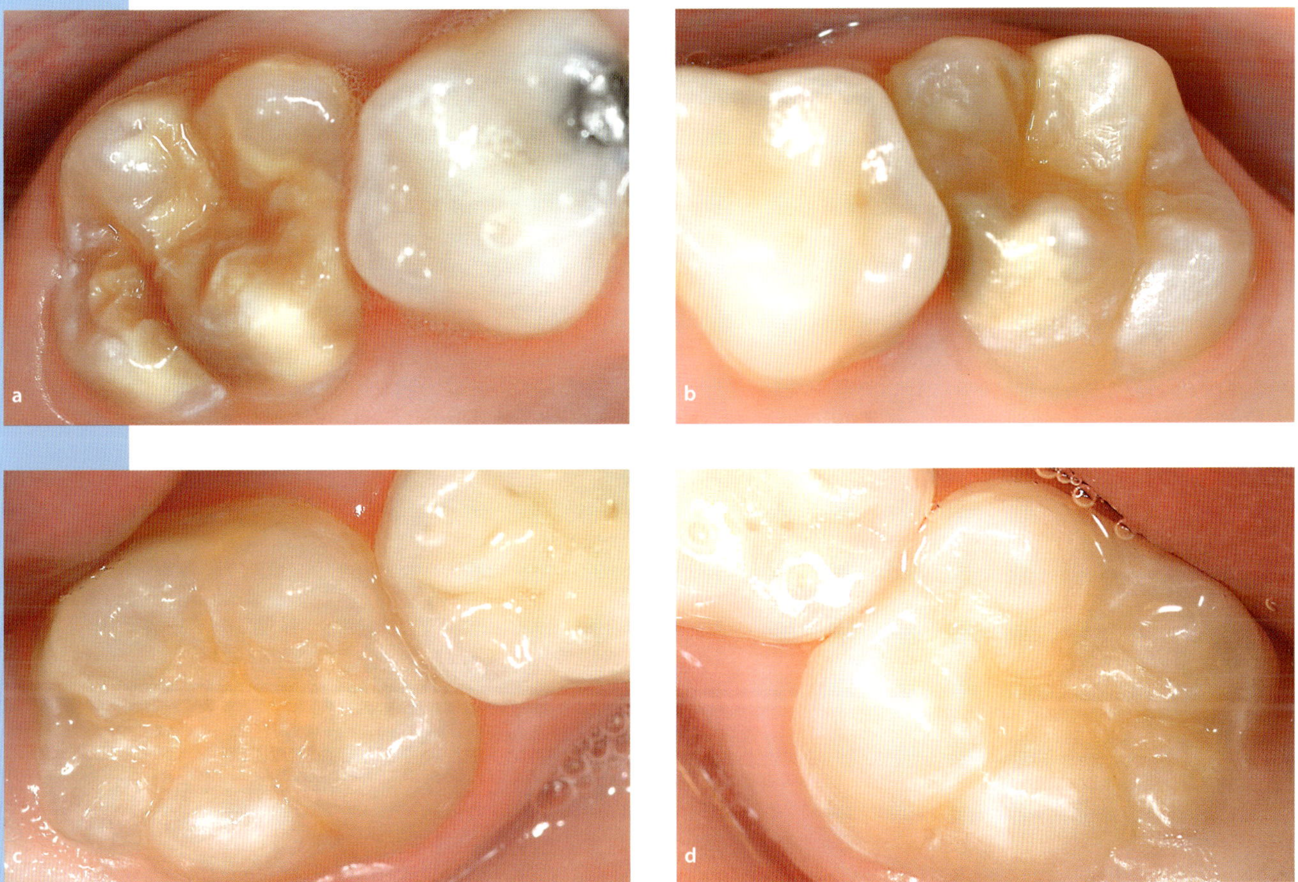

Fig. 2-1a–d A 7-year-old patient with MIH. The first four permanent molars are affected to varying degrees (2-1a 16; 2-1b 26; 2-1c 46; 2-1d 36).

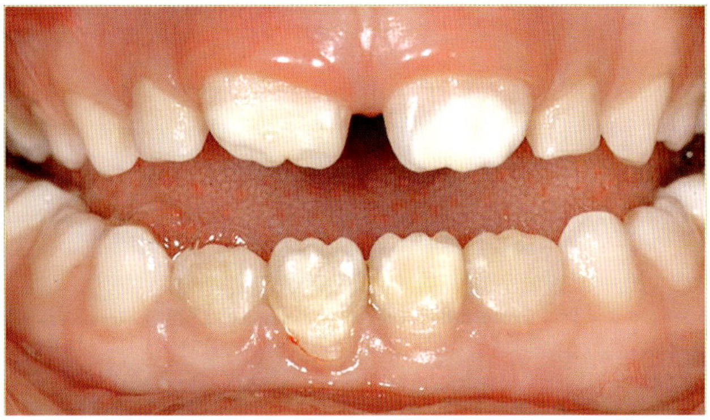

Fig. 2-2 The same patient as in Fig. 2-1. Both the upper and lower incisors are affected.

THE PROBLEM

Jane (age 13) complained about sensitivity to heat and cold in her first molars. The problem was very pronounced during the time maxillary right and left permanent first molars (16, 26) and the mandibular left permanent first molar (36) were erupting. MIH was diagnosed, based on the presence of distinct opacities in these teeth and the breakdown of the enamel. Restorations were placed in the maxillary right and left first molars (16, 26) and in the mandibular left first molar (36) when the patient was 7 years old; these restorations had to be replaced 2 years later. The sensitivity decreased but was not entirely eliminated. On examination it was seen that some of the restoration margins were located in the hypomineralized enamel, and the breakdown of this weakened enamel had led to marginal defects (Figs 2-3a to 2-3d).

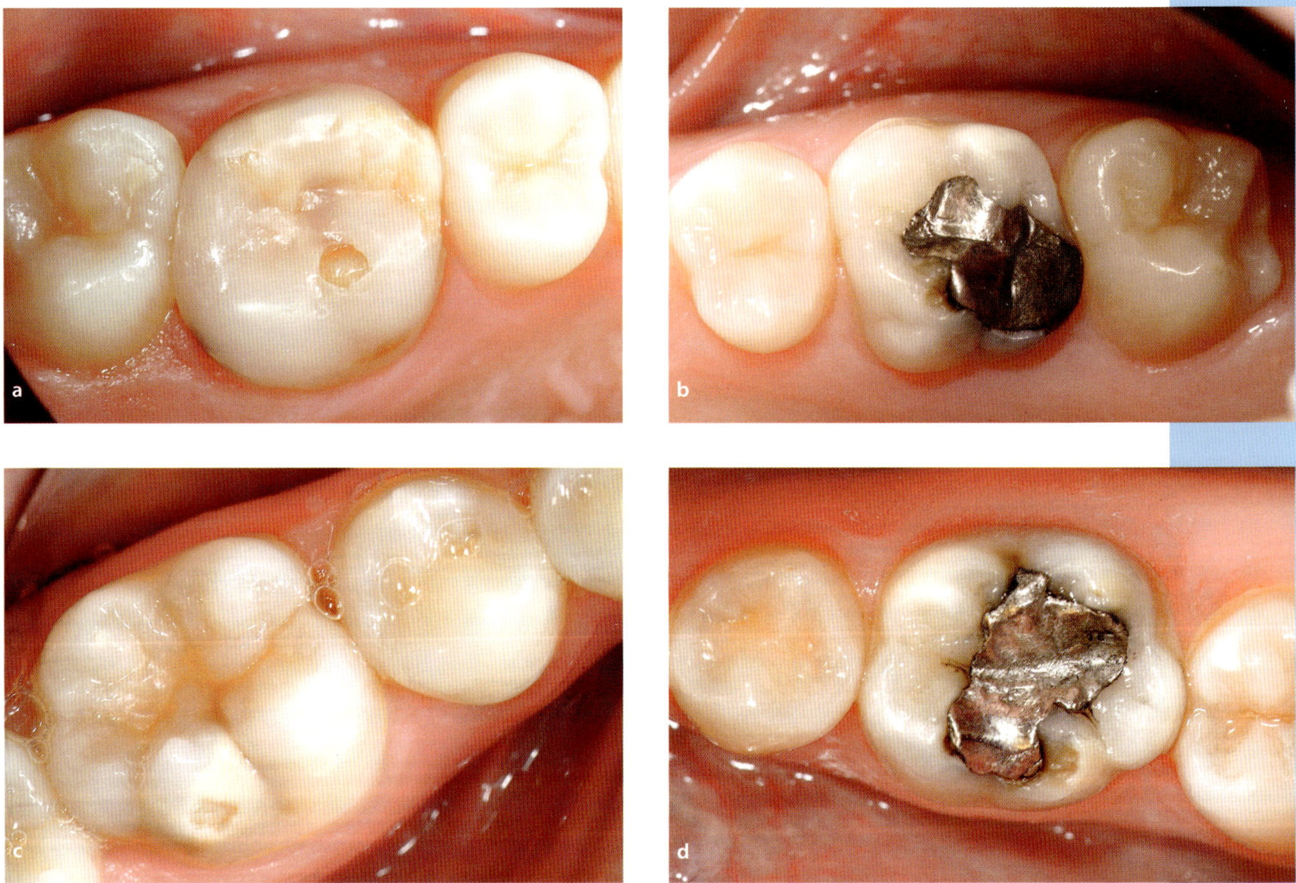

Fig. 2-3a–d At 13 years: the four hypomineralized molars (2-3a 16, 2-3b 26, 2-3c 46, 2-3d 36). The restorations in the maxillary right and left first molars (16, 26) and the mandibular left first molar (36) have an atypical form with margins located in the hypomineralized enamel, resulting in marginal defects in some areas due to breakdown of the weakened enamel.

CASE DESCRIPTION

History

Medical History
ASA I. Jane had experienced repeated ear infections during her first year of life. Antibiotics were prescribed, but the mother did not remember exactly which antibiotics were given. No other medical problems were reported.

Dental History
When Jane was 7 years old, her dentist referred her to the pediatric dentistry department at the University of Leuven because of the presence of hypomineralized molars. As the patient had a fear of dental treatment, the maxillary right and left first molars (16, 26) and the mandibular left first molar (36) were restored under nitrous oxide sedation. This treatment was rather laborious with little cooperation from the patient. The maxillary right and left first molars (16, 26) were restored with compomer and the mandibular left first molar (36) was restored with amalgam. A recall visit was organized every 6 months. The sensitivity decreased but was not eliminated. A highly concentrated fluoride varnish (Duraphat®, Colgate®) was applied to the teeth at each checkup visit. Two years later, the restorations failed and re-treatment was indicated. A decision was made to replace the restorations under general anesthesia. Due to the extensive damage, the maxillary right first molar (16) was restored with a composite (cusp replacement) and the other teeth (26 distal-occlusal-palatal, 36 occlusal-buccal) were restored with amalgam. The annual checkup revealed that the restored teeth remained sensitive to heat and cold. When Jane was 13, owing to more frequent checkups she was comfortable with the idea of having new restorations of these teeth in the dentist's chair under local anesthesia.

Oral Hygiene
In the initial period (ages 7–12 years), Jane's oral hygiene was not good. She avoided brushing her first molars owing to the sensitivity. At each checkup, she was given oral hygiene instructions and the parents were asked to supervise her during brushing. By the time the patient was 13, her oral hygiene had improved markedly.

Examination

The existing restorations in the maxillary right and left first molars (16, 26) and the mandibular left first molar (36) had an atypical form (see Fig. 2-3). The restoration margins are located in the hypomineralized enamel in several areas. In some areas this was accompanied by the presence of marginal defects. Tooth 46 had not been treated and showed creamy white discoloration in the occlusal third of the buccal surface. A flake of enamel had broken off in the middle of this spot. All teeth were sensitive to air from the air syringe. The patient's anterior teeth were not affected and the teeth were otherwise free of caries.

Additional Investigations

The panoramic radiograph taken when Jane was 7 showed enamel defects in the maxillary right and left first molars (16, 26; Fig. 2-4). The bitewing radiographs taken at the checkup visit when she was 13 revealed a radiolucency under the restoration on the distal aspect of the maxillary left first molar (26), and also an enamel defect in the mandibular right first molar (46) (Figs 2-5a, 2-5b).

> **Key Message**
> *If existing restorations in permanent or primary molars have an atypical form, the diagnosis of MIH should be considered.*

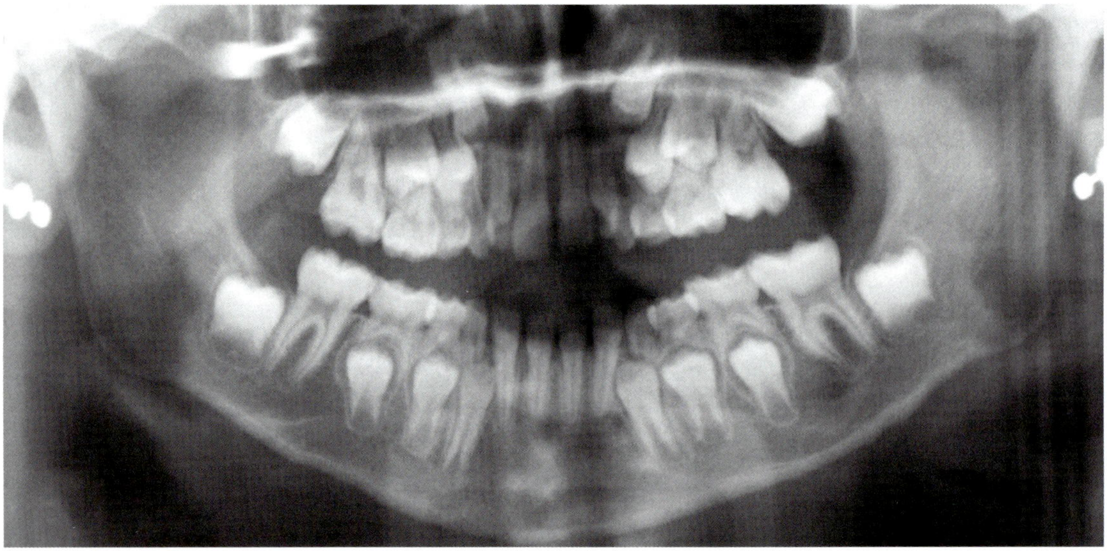

Fig. 2-4 Panoramic radiograph at age 7 shows enamel hypomineralization in the maxillary right and left first molars (16, 26).

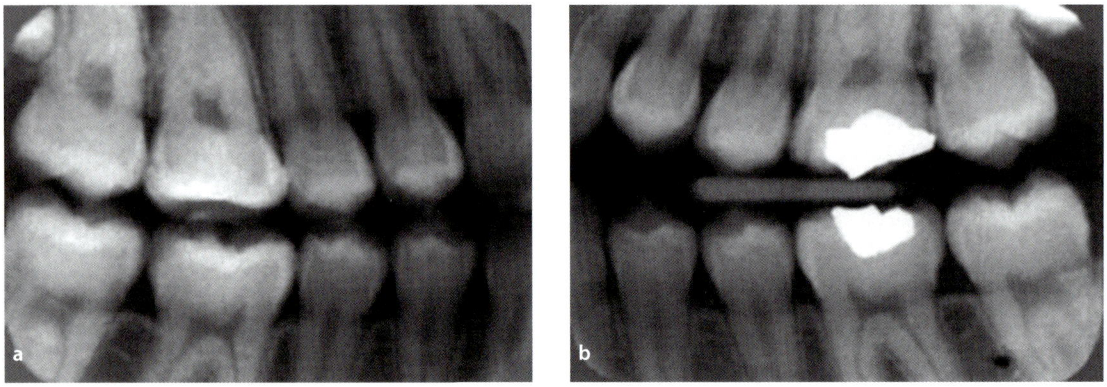

Fig. 2-5a,b Bitewing radiographs at age 13 (2-5a right, 2-5b left). The mandibular right first molar (46) shows enamel hypomineralization, and there is a radiolucency distally under the composite filling in the maxillary right first molar (16).

TREATMENT AIMS

The aim of the treatment was lasting and painless restoration of the hypomineralized molars with resin composite. As Jane had normal occlusion with no need for orthodontic treatment, it was desirable to preserve these teeth.

TREATMENT OPTIONS

Definitive

- Composite restoration of the four first molars.

Alternatives

- The use of nickel-chromium crowns is a good alternative for (temporary) preservation of hypomineralized molars.

Rationale

Restoration of hypomineralized molars is a considerable challenge for the practitioner for various reasons. These teeth are often difficult to anesthetize and first molars are difficult to access in young patients. Therefore, the result of the treatment depends largely on the cooperation of the patient.

Clinical studies have shown that, over a period of 3–4 years, children with hypomineralized molars visit the dentist more frequently than children without molar defects.[2,3] Each hypomineralized molar had to be restored repeatedly due to marginal breakdown or failure of the restoration due to other reasons. Because of difficulties with local anesthesia, children with MIH exhibit difficult behavior during re-treatment and are at increased risk of becoming afraid of the dentist. This problem had occurred in our patient.

Key Message
Restoration of hypomineralized molars with amalgam is not very favourable because it requires fairly invasive retentive cavity preparation, particularly if the weakened enamel is included in the preparation. If the restoration margins are placed in the weakened enamel, the enamel in these areas is most likely to break down over time.

A composite restoration provides the longest-lasting solution, but the procedure is very technique sensitive. Effective removal of all the hypomineralized enamel is required to achieve a reliable bond between the composite and the tooth tissue.[4,5] This cannot always be achieved at the chairside, particularly when the tooth is difficult to anesthetize and in young children. In such patients, sedation or general anesthesia is required to be able to place the most painless and long-lasting composite restorations.

The use of nickel-chromium crowns is accompanied by (excessive) sacrifice of tissue. This also affects future treatment options. For Jane, plastic restoration materials were chosen.

TREATMENT AND FOLLOW-UP

Treatment

The old restorations in the maxillary right and left first molars (16, 26) and the mandibular left first molar (36) were removed along with the remaining hypomineralized enamel. All cavity margins were beveled.

In the mandibular right first molar (46), the white opacity was removed from the buccal aspect, and the occlusal groove was widened to seal the fissure (Figs 2-6a to 2-6d). The local anesthetic worked well during the various restorative sessions, as a result of which the patient remained calm. Isolation was achieved with a metal automatrix (Dentsply), secured with wooden wedges and cotton rolls. A three-step etch-and-rinse adhesive (Optibond Fl, Kerr) was used.[6] The composite restoration was placed in layers using a small-particle hybrid resin composite (Z100, 3M Espe) (Figs 2-7a to 2-7d). The wear resistance of this composite is similar to that of the natural tooth tissue and it has a filler content of more than 60 volume percent, which has adequate strength to withstand the occlusal forces.[7]

Posttreatment Evaluation/Follow-up

Two years later, Jane's restorations are still functioning optimally (Figs 2-8a to 2-8d, Figs 2-9a, 2-9b). Such restorations must be checked on a regular basis and adjustments made if necessary to guarantee the maximal lifespan. If a more permanent restoration of these teeth is desired, an adhesive onlay can be used, made of porcelain or composite.

DISCUSSION

The prevalence of MIH is between 4% and 25%.[8] The cause of this enamel defect is still unclear; infectious diseases during the first 3 years of life, environmental factors, vaccinations, etc., are regarded as possible etiological factors.[9,10] The treatment of hypomineralized molars should preferably take place in several steps. Prevention plays a key role in the management of MIH, with the aim of slowing down the enamel breakdown and preventing development of caries.

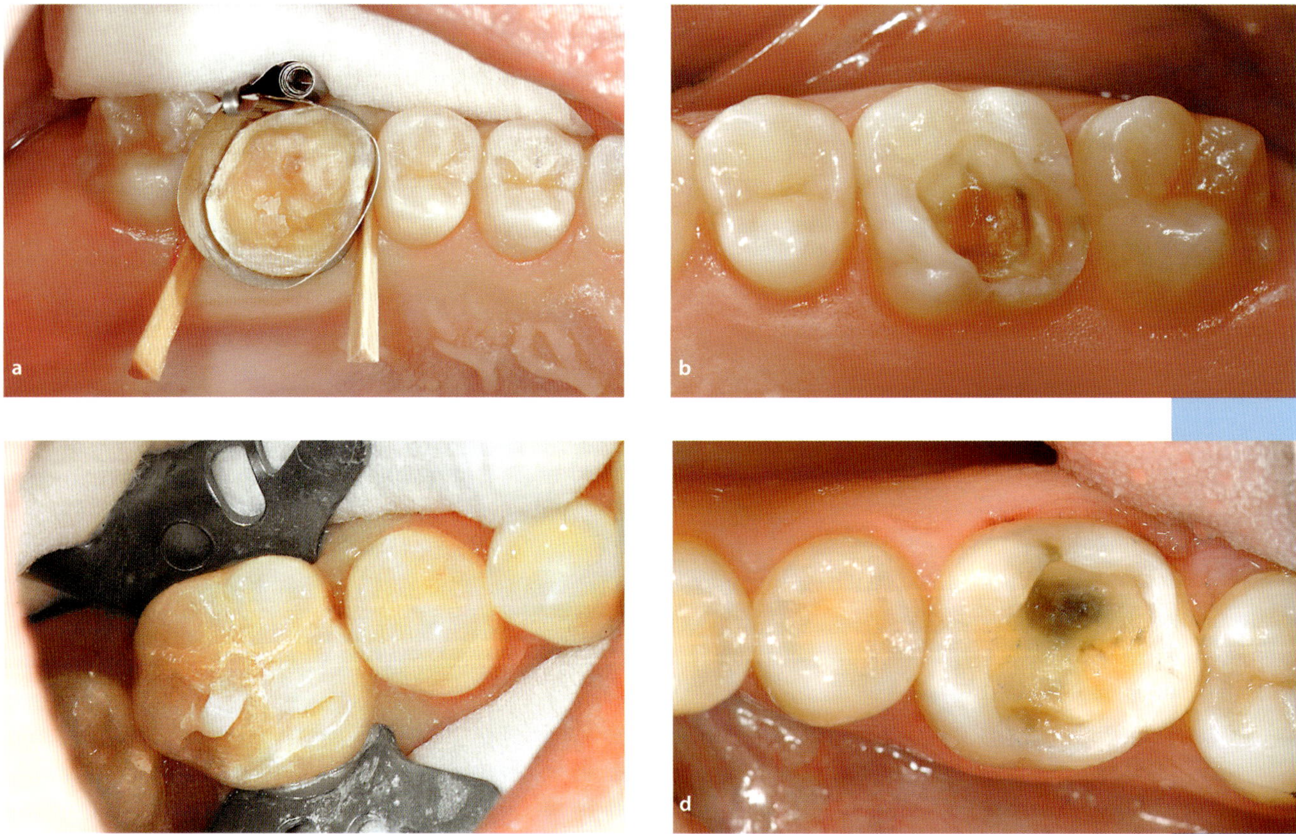

Fig. 2-6a–d Cavity preparation for placement of composite restorations in the four hypomineralized molars. All the hypomineralized enamel was removed. The maxillary right first molar (16) was isolated with a full metal matrix band, secured with wooden wedges and cotton rolls (2-6a 16, 2-6b 26, 2-6c 46, 2-6d 36).

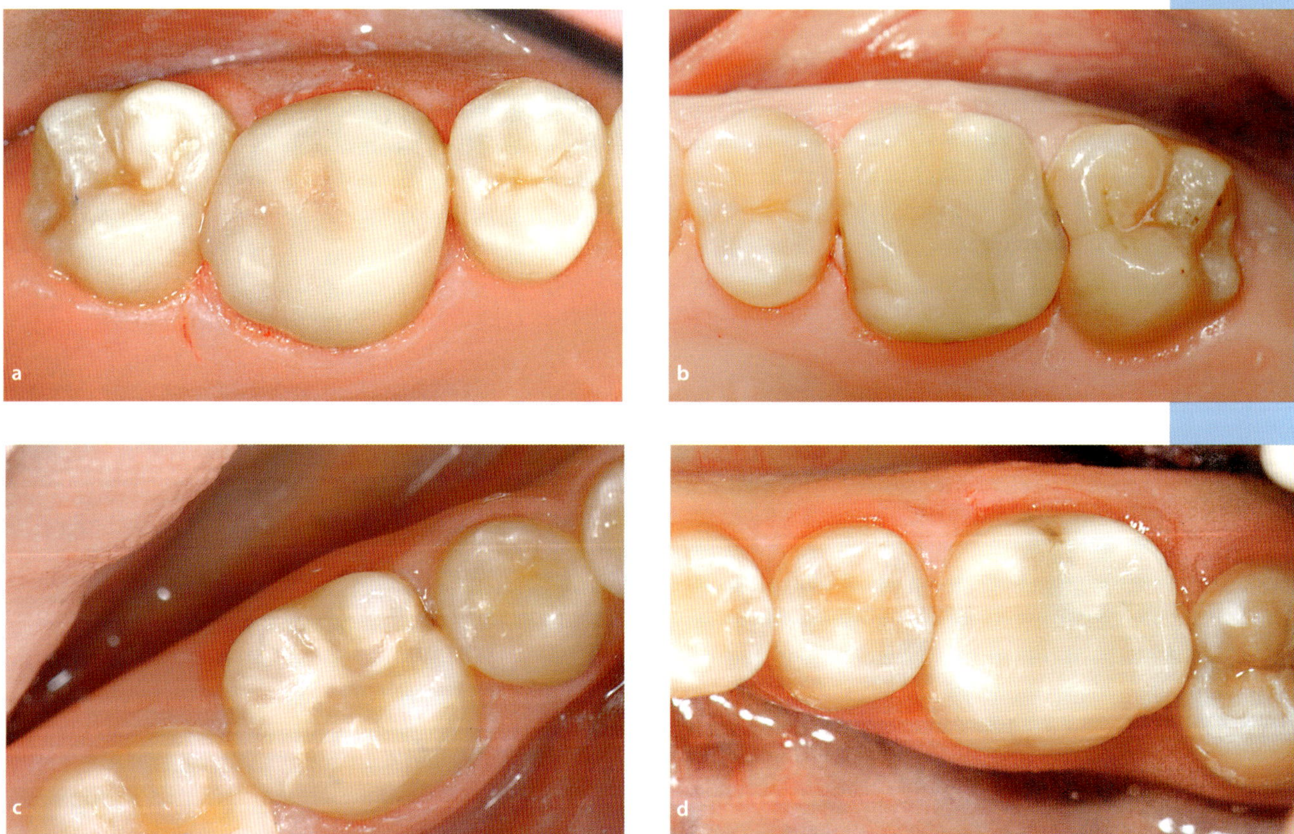

Fig. 2-7a–d The composite restorations in the four hypomineralized molars following placement (2-7a 16, 2-7b 26, 2-7c 46, 2-7d 36).

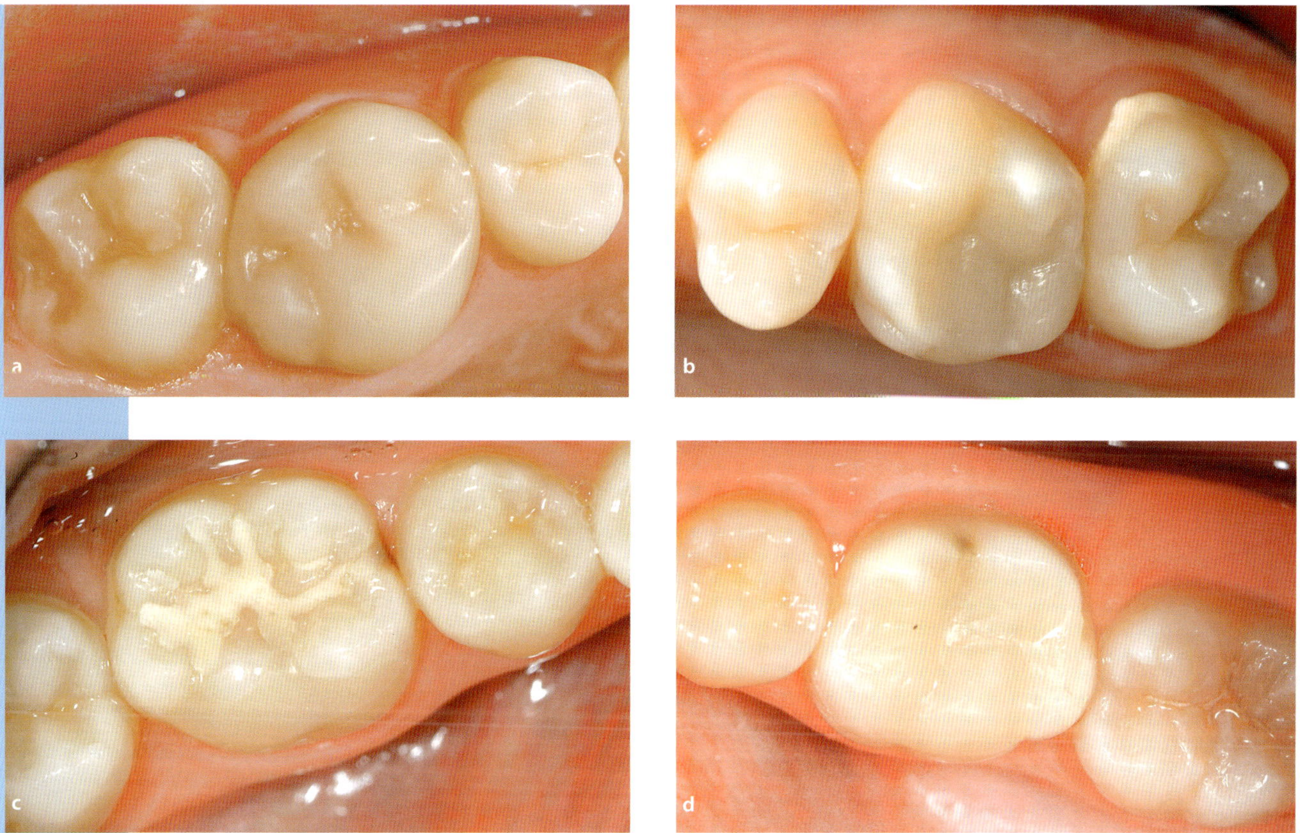

Fig. 2-8a–d Two-year checkup of Jane's composite restorations. All restorations were functioning optimally (2-8a 16, 2-8b 26, 2-8c 46, 2-8d 36).

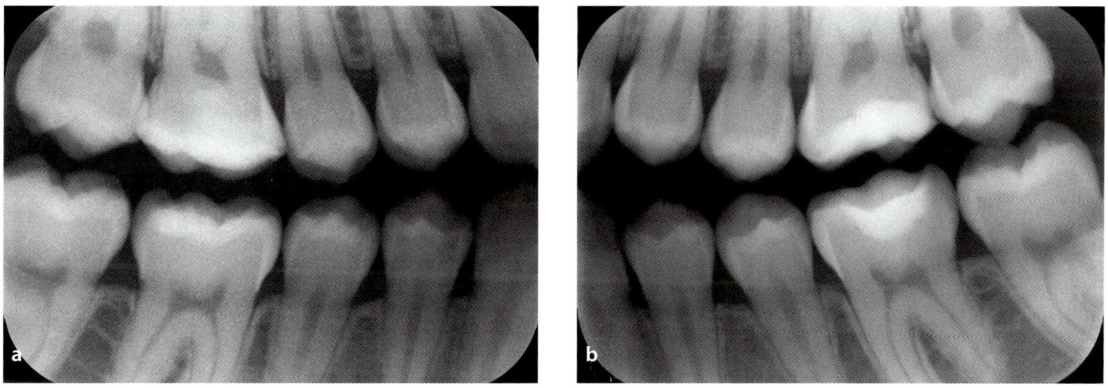

Fig. 2-9a,b Bitewing radiographs also taken 2 years after the placement of the composite restorations (2-9a right, 2-9b left).

The first step is to assess the risk of defects in the first molars as a result of MIH before eruption. This can be done by taking a thorough medical history with specific questions on illnesses and other health problems up to the third year of life. It is also important to keep the first molars under close observation during their eruption. In the case of imminent defects, the patient should be examined every 3 months. The patient can then be educated about the importance of good cleaning with a fluoride toothpaste. Parents' cooperation is essential in this. In addition, the practitioner should attempt to achieve desensitization of the hypomineralized teeth by monthly, local application of a highly concentrated fluoride varnish (eg, Duraphat). Finally, it is important that the patient cuts back on sugary and acidic foods.

Once the first permanent molars have erupted sufficiently, they will have to be sealed as soon as possible. If caries is already detected in the dentin at this stage, restorative treatment must be provided immediately. If a local anesthetic does not have a sufficient analgesic effect, the use of intraosseous anesthesia (eg, Stabident, Fairfax Dental Inc.), should be considered.

Extraction should be considered in very severe cases. Optimal timing of the extraction is advisable, so that the second and third molars can erupt in a more mesial position and close the extraction space. It is best to do this in consultation with an orthodontist, and extractions are usually done once the development of the bifurcation area of the root of the distal tooth has started.

Restorations should be performed as painlessly as possible and with the aim of lasting as long as possible. Effective removal of all the hypomineralized tissue is essential to achieve a lasting composite restoration. In addition, composite restorations should be placed in layers using a small-particle hybrid composite and a reliable adhesive system.

REFERENCES

1. Weerheijm KL, Jalevik B, Alaluusua S. Molar–incisor hypomineralization. Caries Res 2001;35:390–391.
2. Jälevik B, Klingberg GA. Dental treatment, dental fear and behaviour management problems in children with severe enamel hypomineralization of their permanent first molars. Int J Paediatr Dent 2002;12:24–32.
3. Kotsanos N, Kaklamanos EG, Arapostathis K. Treatment management of first permanent molars in children with Molar-Incisor Hypomineralisation. Eur J Paediatr Dent 2005;6:179–184.
4. Jälevik B, Dietz W, Norèn JG. Scanning electron micrograph analysis of hypomineralized enamel in permanent first molars. Int J Paediatr Dent 2005;15:233–40.
5. William V, Burrow MF, Palamara JEA, Messer LB. Microshear bond strength of resin composite to teeth affected by molar hypomineralization using 2 adhesive systems. Pediatr Dent 2006;28:233–241.
6. Van Meerbeek B, De Munck J, Yoshida Y, Inoue S, Vargas M, Vijay P, et al. Buonocore memorial lecture. Adhesion to enamel and dentin: current status and future challenges. Oper Dent 2003;28:215–235.
7. Willems G, Lambrechts P, Braem M, Celis JP, Vanherle G. A classification of dental composites according to their morphological and mechanical characteristics. Dent Mater 1992;8:310–319.
8. William V, Messer LB, Burrow MF. Molar incisor hypomineralization: review and recommendations for clinical management. Pediatr Dent 2006;28:224–232.
9. Beentjes VEVM, Weerheijm KL, Groen HJ. [Factors involved in the aetiology of hypomineralized first permanent molars.] [Article in Dutch] Ned Tijdschr Tandheelkd 2002;109:387–90.
10. Jälevik B, Norèn JG, Klingberg G, Barregård L. Etiologic factors influencing the prevalence of demarcated opacities in permanent first molars in a group of Swedish children. Eur J Oral Sci 2001;109:230–234.

3

Dentinogenesis Imperfecta Type II

Satu Alaluusua
Heikki Alapulli

Key words: dentinogenesis imperfecta

Age category: 7–12 years

Definition

Inherited dentin defects have traditionally been classified as dentinogenesis imperfecta types I (DI-I), II (DI-II), and III (DI-III), and dentin dysplasia types I (DD-I) and II (DD-II).[1] DI-II, DI-III, and DD-II have been viewed as a continuum of defects and accordingly they have been mapped to the same region in chromosome 4 and associated with defects in the dentin sialophosphoprotein (*DSPP*) gene.[2]

The most common of the inherited dentin diseases is DI-II with the estimated incidence of 1:8000.[3] DI-II is an autosomal dominant disorder with generally complete penetrance and a low frequency of *de novo* mutations.[1,3] It affects both the primary and the permanent dentitions. The primary teeth are more severely affected than the permanent teeth. Characteristic features of the teeth are: blue-gray or amber brown opalescent color; bulbous, cervically constricted crowns, short roots, and early obliteration of the pulp chambers and root canals. Histologically, the dentinal tubules are sparse and irregular. Under occlusal stress, the enamel cracks readily and the exposed dentin undergoes severe attrition.

THE PROBLEM

John (age 12) is affected with DI-II. His permanent teeth have just erupted and there is a need to cover these teeth with crowns. If the treatment is postponed, severe attrition will take place with all the consequences, such as deepening of the bite and advancing problems in achieving retention for the prosthetic crowns. Furthermore, the amber color of the teeth is eye-catching.

CASE DESCRIPTION

History

Medical History

ASA I. John had been in good health and his medical history was non-contributory. The family history supported the diagnosis of DI-II; John came from a big family where the disease could be traced back several generations. A previous study had shown that the affected family members had a mutation in the *DSPP* gene in the third nucleotide before exon 3 in intron 2.[4] *DSPP* codes for dentin sialophosphoprotein, which after translation splits into dentin sialoprotein, an essential protein for the mineralization of dentin, and dentin phosphoprotein.5 The mutation in the patient's family was in the dentin sialoprotein coding part of *DSPP*.

Dental History

All primary teeth had a yellowish-brown, opalescent appearance (Fig. 3-1a). Already at the age of 3 years, John had severe attrition (Figs 3-1b, 3-1c) with an anterior open bite. The left maxillary molars were infected and had been treated with pulpotomy, but without success. These teeth had to be extracted. To establish proper vertical dimension and to prevent further occlusal wear and pulpal involvement, extractions and space loss, at the age of 3 years and 9 months, the rest of the primary molars were covered with stainless steel crowns (SSCs; 3M ESPE, Seefeld, Germany) under general anesthesia.

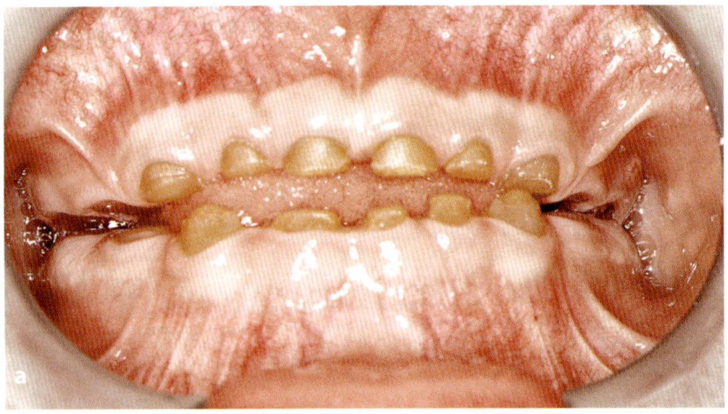

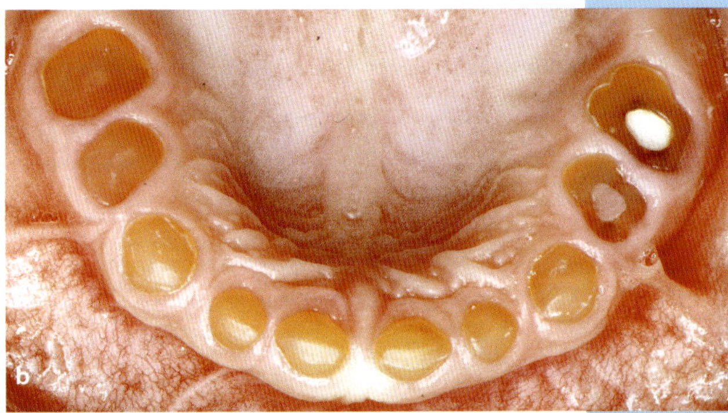

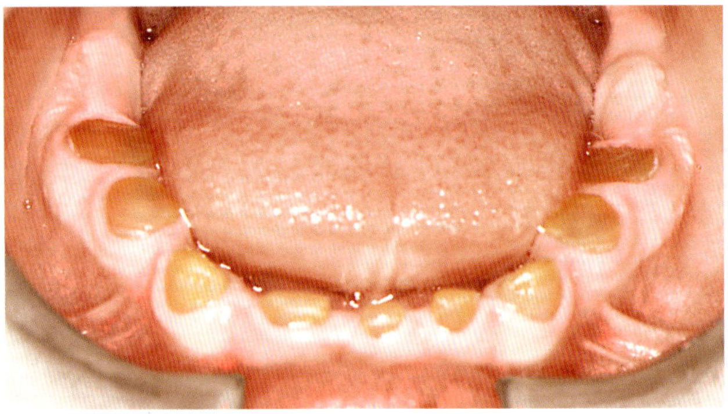

Fig. 3-1a The typical amber colour of primary teeth with DI-II.

Fig. 3-1b At the age of 3 years, severe attrition of the upper molars had resulted in exposure of the pulps of the maxillary left primary first and second molars (64, 65).

Fig. 3-1c Severe attrition is also seen in the lower molars.

Due to severe attrition, the patient's molars had a different crown shape from that of the preformed SCCs. After reducing the height of the SSCs with scissors, gingival constriction of the crowns had to be done. We made four slits (mesiobuccal, mesiopalatal, distobuccal, distopalatal) at the gingival end of the crown. We then overlapped the two parts of each slit surface of the crown and point-welded the parts together. The gingival margins were further crimped with pliers. In this way better mechanical retention was achieved and the gingival adaptation of the SCCs became acceptable. After final shaping and polishing, the crowns were cemented with glass-ionomer cement. The primary incisors and canines were not covered.

Key Message

To prevent occlusal wear and pulpal involvement, covering the primary molars with SSC as early as possible may be necessary.

At the age of 6 years, the patient's permanent first molars had erupted sufficiently for the placement of SSCs. The crowns were placed under local anesthesia and nitrous oxide sedation. A panoramic radiograph taken at the age of 9 years revealed that the pulps and the root canals of the permanent first molars and incisors were totally, or for the most part, obliterated (Fig. 3-2).

There were no apparent problems with John's speech or mastication. He had bruxism, and restoration of the permanent incisors with resin composite was discussed with the child and the parent, but it was decided to postpone this treatment.

Examination

At the age of 11 years and 8 months, the second molars, canines, and premolars (except the maxillary left second premolar) had erupted (Figs 3-3a to 3-3c). There was a lack of space for the unerupted maxillary left second premolar and it was decided that the tooth would be extracted later. There

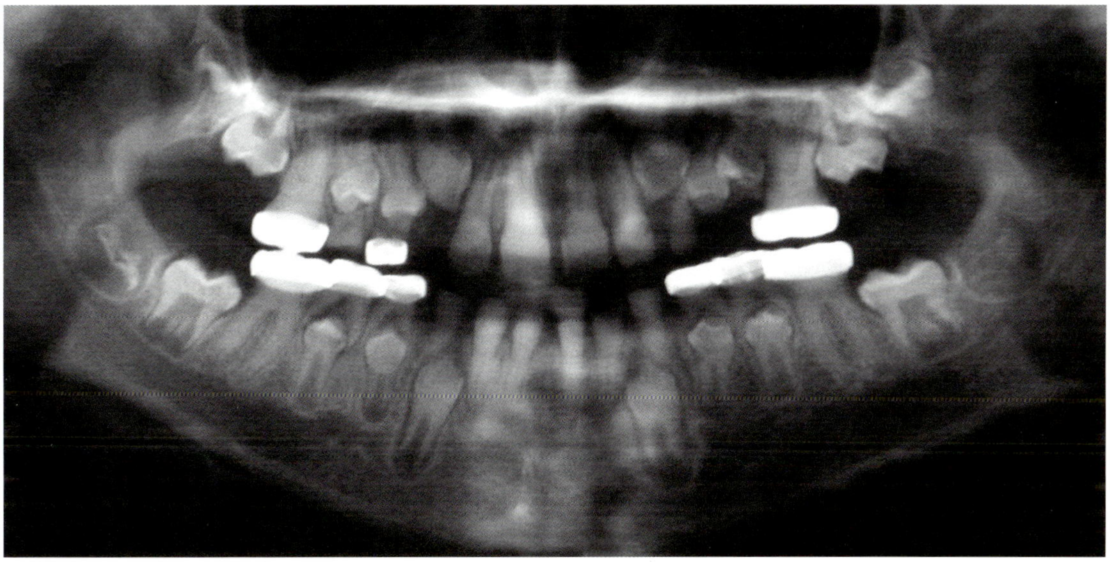

Fig. 3-2 Panoramic radiograph taken at the age of 9 years shows pulpal and root canal obliteration in permanent first molars and incisors. Obliteration of the pulps is also seen in the developing teeth.

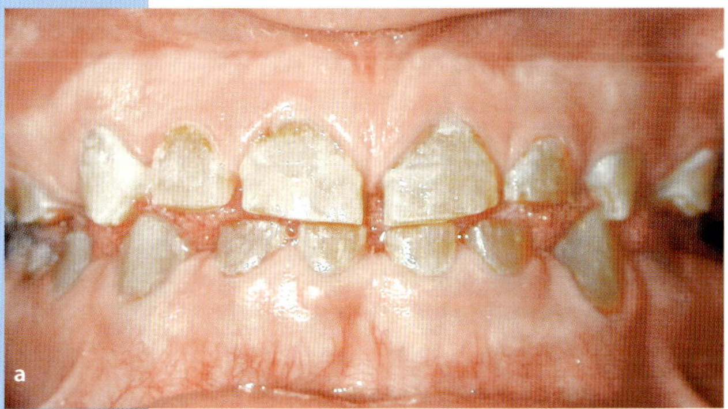

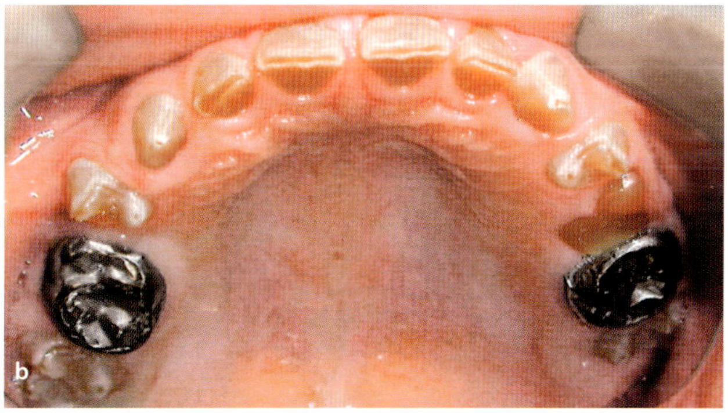

Fig. 3-3a Amber-colored erupting mandibular permanent incisors.

Fig. 3-3b,c Attrition already present in the newly erupted permanent first molars.

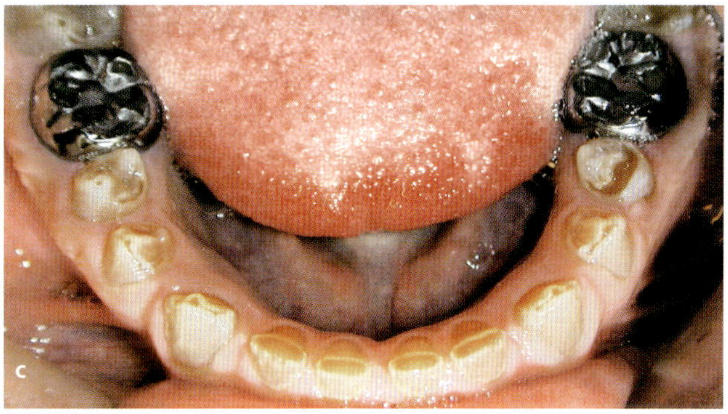

was some attrition in the newly erupted teeth and in the incisors. The overbite and overjet were both nearly 0 mm. The oral hygiene was good.

TREATMENT AIM

The aim of the treatment was esthetically and functionally acceptable rehabilitation of the dentition, allowing normal growth.

TREATMENT OPTIONS

Definitive

- Laboratory-made composite crown coverage for the incisors, canines, and premolars, and SSC coverage for the molars.

Alternatives

- Polycarbonate or laboratory-made all-ceramic crown coverage of the incisors, canines, and premolars and SSCs or gold crowns/onlays in the molar region.

Rationale

Material selection for crown coverage of the permanent teeth is challenging, since the crowns should last for several years but the costs still have to be reasonable. In the present case, laboratory-made fiber-reinforced composite crowns were preferred for the incisors, canines, and premolars. These crowns are esthetically acceptable but cheaper than prosthetic crowns and still resist abrasion and breakdown fairly well. SSCs were preferred in the molar region since they are technically easier to make than prosthetic crowns at the age when the gingival margin level is still high.

TREATMENT AND FOLLOW-UP

Treatment

Preparation of permanent teeth with DI-II is difficult because of the limited and defective hard tissues of the crown of the teeth. The abnormal tubular structure, decreased mineral content, and presence of fewer crystals in the dentin are likely to weaken the shear bond strength of resin composites. Furthermore, cracked enamel gives poor support for adhesion. Therefore, replacement of some composite crowns was expected. It is important to inform the child and the parents of the prognosis. We expect to fit prosthetic crowns in the molar area in 5 years time. Due to age-related gingival recession, which would expose the amber-coloured hard tissue, the composite crowns on the incisors and canines would need to be replaced within 5–15 years.

The patient's treatment was started by placement of the laboratory-made composite crowns on the mandibular premolars. Shoulder preparations were extended to the gingival margin. Occlusally about 1 mm of the crown was reduced. Since only minor occlusal preparation was possible, increase in occlusal height was expected. This was not a problem in the present case, but it required replace-

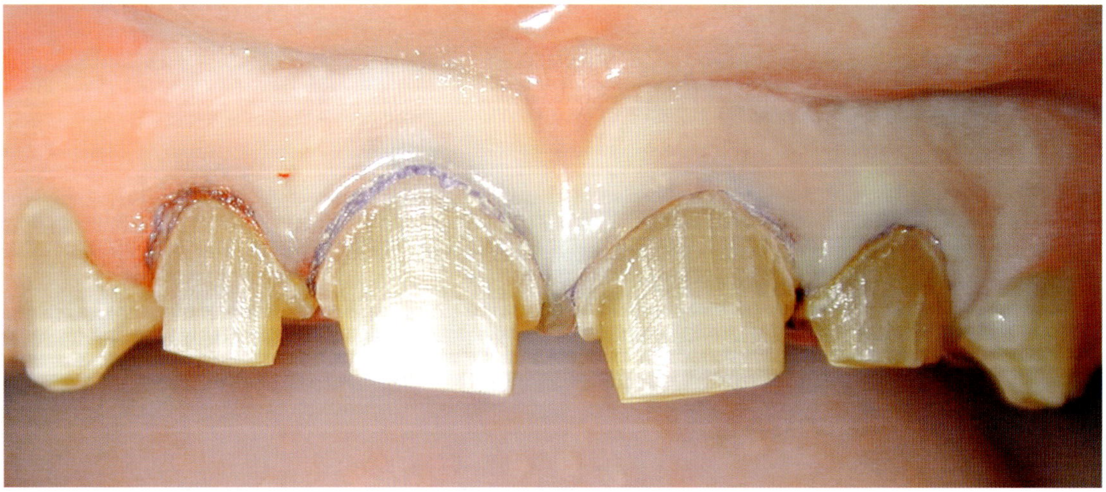

Fig. 3-4 Shoulder preparation in the maxillary incisors. Blue retraction cord is seen in the gingival sulci.

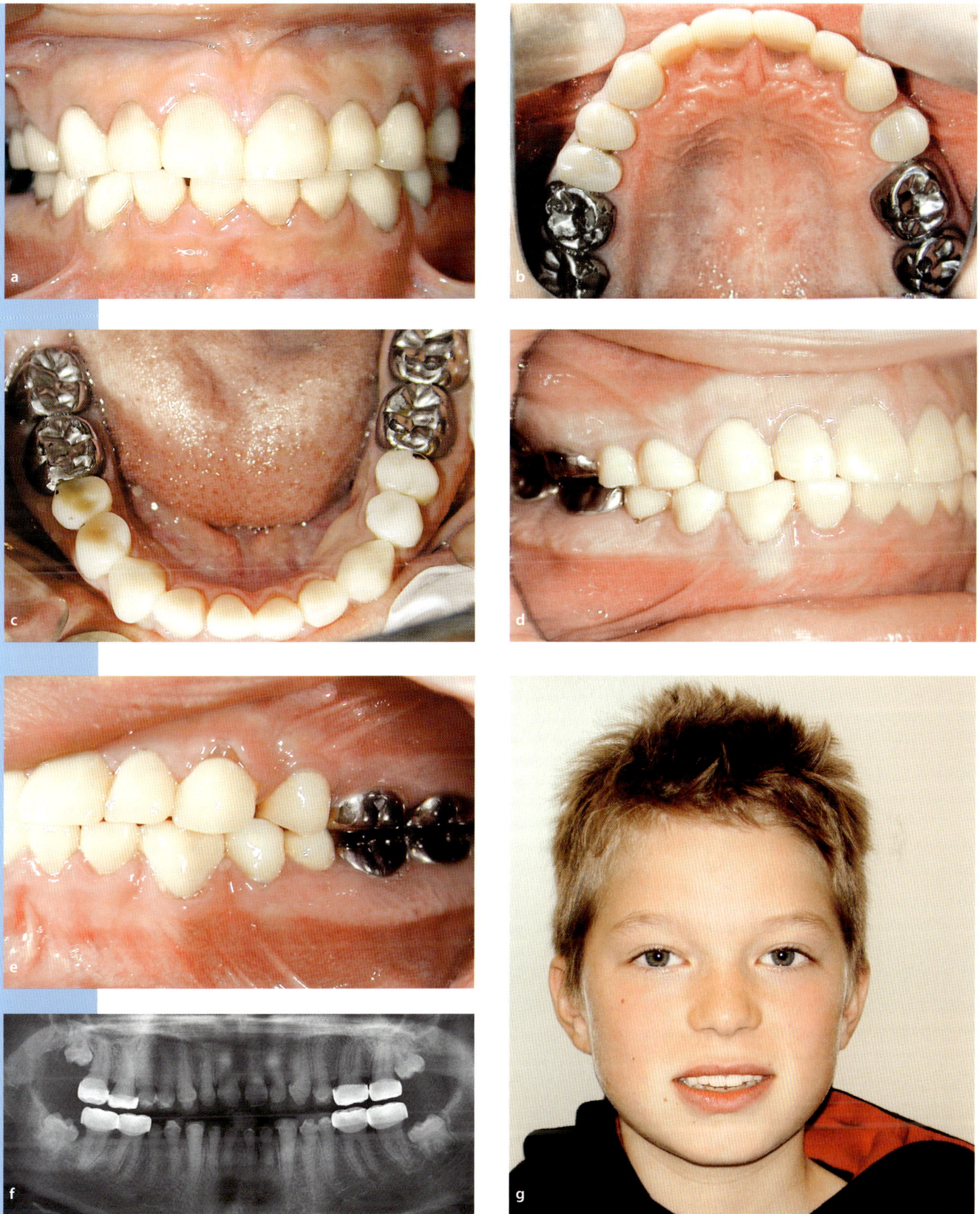

Fig. 3-5a–g Completed treatment with composite crowns on the anterior teeth and premolars, and SSC on the molars, at the age of 12 years. The panoramic radiograph reveals total or almost total obliteration of the root canals in all teeth except the third molars. Poor adaptation of the stainless steel crowns on the mandibular second molars may hinder eruption of the third molars (38, 48).

ment of the SSCs on the first molars, too, to balance the occlusion. The laboratory-made composite crowns (GC Corporation, Tokyo, Japan) were reinforced with a fiber net (Stick Tech Corporation, Turku, Finland). The crowns were cemented with a resin composite cement (Panavia F, Kuraray, Tokyo, Japan). The placement of the crowns at each appointment was done symmetrically to distribute the occlusal stresses evenly.

The next step was the placement of laboratory-made composite crowns on the maxillary incisors and SSCs on the lower second molars. Figure 3-4 shows the shoulder preparation prior to crown placement in the incisor region. The treatment was completed with crowning of the rest of the teeth by the age of 12 years (Figs 3-5a to 3-5g). However, within 12 months, the crowns of the lower canines and the mandibular right second premolar (45) had broken. We believe that this was partly due to bruxism and partly due to the under-preparation of the tooth crown and subsequently too thin composite layer. The crowns were redone with more extensive preparation and an occlusal splint was introduced. The upper left second premolar was extracted by a flap operation at the age of 13 years. Occlusion was normal and adaptation of the composite crowns was good. On the contrary, the poor marginal adaptation of the distal parts of the SCCs in the lower second molars may prevent eruption of the wisdom teeth.

Posttreatment Evaluation/Follow-up

Three of the composite crowns fractured soon after placement. However, no further problems were evident on further recall appointments in the next 2.5 years. Future follow-up visits were planned once a year. The eruption of the third molars is being followed on panoramic radiographs.

> ***Key Message***
> *Dental treatment of DI-II is lifelong. Regular follow-up is essential and treatment, such as replacement of fractured crowns, should be done without delay in order to prevent further problems.*

DISCUSSION

Several mutations of the *DSPP* gene have been found, and the clinical manifestations in the teeth depend on the alteration of the biochemical nature of the downstream protein sequence. There is a wide range of phenotypical features among affected families and the management is matched to the clinical expression of the disease. For example, in some families the prominent feature is severe attrition, as in our patient's family, causing problems in occlusion and increasing risk of pulpal exposure. In other families, apical periodontitis may be common in both the primary and permanent teeth, with only minor attrition and no obvious pulpal exposure.[6] For individual treatment planning, it is invaluable to know the characteristics of the condition within the patient's family.

Children with DI-II need more dental treatment than children with normal teeth. The treatment starts early in life. When severe attrition is expected, it is wise to protect the primary first molars once they have erupted with SCCs as suggested by Sapir and Shapira.[7] Because of the general lack of cooperation at an early age, general anesthesia is required at the first stage and probably also at the second stage when the primary second molars erupt. However, in later stages of treatment, general anesthesia is rarely needed, although the long treatment sessions require much patience from the child. John's primary molars were treated under general anesthesia and the permanent teeth were treated under local anesthesia.

CONCLUSION

Dental treatment of DI-II is lifelong. It requires active involvement from the patient, the parents, and the dentist. In addition to rehabilitation of the occlusion with the help of crowns, caries prevention is important, as well as an orthodontic evaluation.[8] In order to improve the esthetic appearance at an early age, crown coverage of the primary incisors and canines and newly erupted permanent incisors should be considered. In our patient, we feel that we should have been more active in covering these teeth earlier.

The treatment as a whole is time-consuming and often expensive, but not always successful. We have found that if a child has bruxism, occlusal splinting may prevent attrition and fracture of the crowns. Long-term reports from experienced clinicians on treatment techniques and materials used are needed to develop optimal treatment strategies.

REFERENCES

1. Shields ED, Bixler D, el-Kafrawy AM. A proposed classification for heritable human dentine defects with a description of a new entity. Arch Oral Biol 1973;18:543–553.
2. McKnight DA, Hart PS, Hart TC, Hartsfield JK, Wilson A, Wright JT, et al. A comprehensive analysis of normal variation and disease-causing mutations in the human *DSPP* gene. Hum Mutat 2008;29:1392–1340.
3. Witkop CJ, Rao S. Inherited Defects in Tooth Structure. Baltimore: Williams & Wilkins, 1971:153.
4. Holappa H, Nieminen P, Tolva L, Lukinmaa PL, Alaluusua S. Splicing site mutations in dentin sialophosphoprotein causing dentinogenesis imperfecta type II. Eur J Oral Sci 2006;114:381–384.
5. MacDougall M, Simmons D, Luan X, Nydegger J, Feng J, Gu TT. Dentin phosphoprotein and dentin sialoprotein are cleavage products expressed from a single transcript coded by a gene on human chromosome 4. Dentin phosphoprotein DNA sequence determination. J Biol Chem 1997;272:835–842.
6. Malmgren B, Lindskog S, Elgadi A, Norgren S. Clinical, histopathologic, and genetic investigation in two large families with dentinogenesis imperfecta type II. Hum Genet 2004;114, 491–498.
7. Sapir S, Shapira J. Dentinogenesis imperfecta: an early treatment strategy. Pediatr Dent 2001;23:232–237.
8. Huth KCH, Paschos E, Sagner T, Hickel R. Diagnostic features and pedodontic-orthodontic management in dentinogenesis imperfecta type II: a case report. Int J Paed Dent 2002;12:316–321.

4

Hypophosphatasia

Anne B. Skaare
Veslemøy E. Bjørkeng
Sven Simonsen
Anne Grethe Myhre
Ivar Espelid

Key words: hypophosphatasia, alkaline phosphatase, premature tooth loss, primary teeth, mineralization

Age category: 0–4 years

Definition

Hypophosphatasia is a rare, inherited metabolic disorder that occurs in four forms. The later the symptoms are manifested, the less severe is the form of the disease present, and the dental findings may be the first and only clinical and radiographic manifestations. Hypophosphatasia is characterized by a deficiency of serum and bone alkaline phosphatase (ALP) activity causing defective bone and altered cementum formation. The disorder is caused by mutations in the liver/bone/kidney alkaline phosphatase (*ALPL*) gene encoding the tissue–non-specific alkaline phosphatase (TNAP) enzyme. When the activity of this enzyme is reduced, the mineralization process is disturbed. The diagnosis is based on reduced serum ALP activity, increased urinary phosphoethanolamine, and DNA sequencing of the *ALPL* gene. The disorder is inherited as either an autosomal recessive or a dominant trait and is highly variable in clinical expression, ranging from premature loss of primary teeth to presence of neonatal death. When the only clinical sign of the disorder is premature loss of fully rooted primary teeth, it is often referred to as odontohypophosphatasia. The anterior teeth are most frequently affected. Marginal bone loss in combination with hypoplastic or aplastic cementum is the reason for the premature tooth loss.

Key Message

As premature tooth loss may be the first clinical sign of odontohypophosphatasia, the pediatric dentist has a key role in early diagnosis of hypophosphatasia.

THE PROBLEM

Two girls and two boys (two of whom were siblings) had each, before the age of 3 years, lost four or more primary anterior teeth without any obvious reason.

CASE DESCRIPTION
CASE 1

History

Medical History

At the time of referral, Agnes had no history of medical problems. She was the first child of the mother and the first child of healthy unrelated parents. The father had two healthy children from a previous marriage.

Dental History

Agnes was referred by her dentist to the department of pediatric dentistry at the University of Oslo, at 22 months of age for premature loss of primary incisors. Her first primary incisors, the maxillary central incisors (71, 81), erupted at 3 months of age. After mild trauma at 9 months, both incisors exfoliated. Before Agnes was 18 months old, she had lost all her mandibular incisors despite little sign of root resorption and no further evident trauma.

Examination

At the first clinical examination in the university department of pediatric dentistry, five primary incisors were missing (four mandibular incisors and the maxillary left central incisor), while the remaining maxillary right primary central incisor (51) was mobile. There was no or only slight gingival inflammation. The second primary molars had not erupted. Small opacities in the enamel of both the primary maxillary lateral incisors (52, 62) were seen. Neither the mother nor the father had experienced premature tooth loss. At the time of examination, the patient had no siblings.

Additional Investigations

Intraoral radiographs revealed horizontal alveolar bone loss of nearly half of the root length in the maxillary anterior region, with widening of the periodontal space. There was no sign of apical root resorption, but an apical root fragment was seen in the region of the left maxillary primary central incisor (61). The pulp chambers were enlarged (Fig. 4-1).

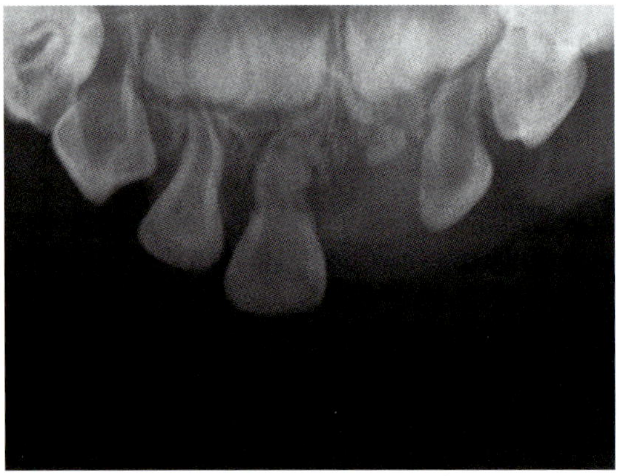

Fig 4-1 Case 1 (22 months). Radiograph shows horizontal bone loss, increased periodontal width and large pulp chambers. Note apical root fragment of the maxillary left central incisor (61).

Agnes was referred for a medical examination with a view to the inherited disorder hypophosphatasia where premature tooth loss may be the first and only clinical sign of the disease.

Laboratory Findings

Blood tests revealed pathologically reduced serum ALP activity, and urinary phosphoethanolamine levels were nearly eight times above the upper limit of normal. Vitamin D status and urinary calcium secretion were normal. Radiographic examination of the base of the hand and thorax was also normal.

Molecular Biology Screening

Screening for mutation in the *ALPL* gene showed that both parents were carriers, and that the patient had inherited one mutation from the father and one from the mother. The mother's mutation was previously described but the father's was not. The parents both had slightly increased urinary phosphoethanolamine levels, indicating carrier condition.

TREATMENT OPTIONS

Definitive

- To schedule individual preventive measures, including professional cleaning and plaque control.
- Observation of primary teeth and early intervention for carious lesions.

- To provide information to the parents about the nature of the disease and to keep in contact with the pediatrician.
- Manage early loss of primary teeth.

Alternatives

- Consider partial dentures in case of loss of primary molars. This may be a good alternative not only from the functional and esthetic viewpoints, but may also prevent migration of teeth.
- Coordinate treatment with other dental specialists such as an orthodontist.

CASE 2

History

Medical History

Peter was Agnes's younger brother and was diagnosed with hypophosphatasia during his first year of life.

Dental History

At 10 months of age, eight primary teeth had erupted, of which the mandibular right primary central incisor (81) was mobile. At 19 months of age the four mandibular incisors had exfoliated, and before the age of 3, the mandibular canines were lost.

Examination

Occlusal caries was registered in both the mandibular primary second molars (75, 85) at the age of 3. The oral hygiene was good, and the gingiva showed no signs of inflammation.

Additional Investigations

Intraoral radiographs revealed horizontal bone loss in the maxillary anterior region and enlarged pulp chambers (Fig. 4-2).

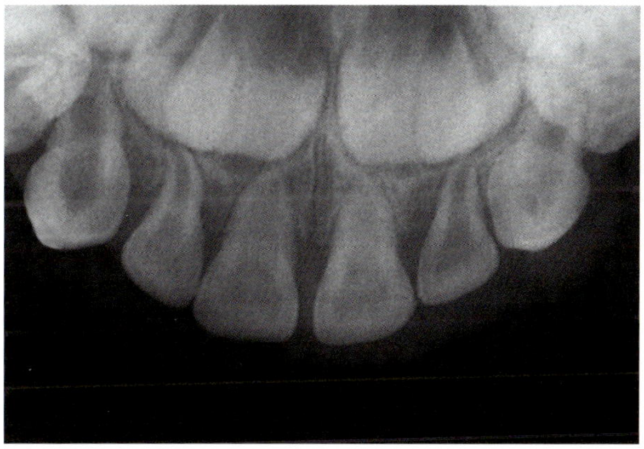

Fig. 4-2 Case 2 (3 years). Radiograph showing enlarged pulp chambers and reduced alveolar bone.

CASE 3

History

Medical History

Stephanie was referred at 19 months of age from the maternal and child healthcare center to the local hospital for delayed motor development. Hematological screening and radiographic examination of the pelvis and hips were normal. Stephanie had been walking independently from 14 months of age, but her gait remained stiff. There was a tendency for stumbling and falling. When she was 26 months old, she was referred to the university hospital for delayed development characterized by waddling and stiff gait. At that time, she also periodically had pain in her feet and knees. A new radiographic examination did not reveal any abnormality, but there was indication of bow legs and delayed development of the musculature. She also had slightly reduced serum calcium levels. She was diagnosed as having hypotonia, and further neurological investigations were planned. Stephanie was the younger of two siblings; an older brother of 15 years was healthy.

Dental History

When Stephanie was 18 months old, both the mandibular central incisors (71, 81) were avulsed, presumably because of stumbling and falling over. But at the age of 2 years, two mandibular incisors had shed. The local dentist associated the tooth loss with the previous trauma, but the mother insisted on being referred to the university hospital.

Examination

Stephanie was referred to the department of pediatric dentistry at the age of 31 months for premature loss of the four mandibular primary incisors (Fig. 4-3a).

The clinical examination revealed in addition, increased mobility of the maxillary left primary central incisor (61), the mandibular left primary canine (73), and the mandibular right primary canine (83). The patient's oral hygiene was good, she was caries-free and there was no gingival inflammation. None of the family members had experienced premature tooth loss.

Additional Investigations

Intraoral radiographs revealed horizontal alveolar bone loss of approximately half of the root length of the upper central incisors and marked alveolar bone loss in the region of the mandibular right primary canine (83). This primary canine was highly mobile and showed delayed root development, with a wide pulp chamber and no sign of apical closure; it finally exfoliated without normal root resorption (Figs 4-3b, 4-3c).

The premature tooth loss in combination with the hypotonic musculature or waddling gait, clearly indicated hypophosphatasia, and Stephanie was referred to the hospital for further investigations with a view toward this inherited disorder.

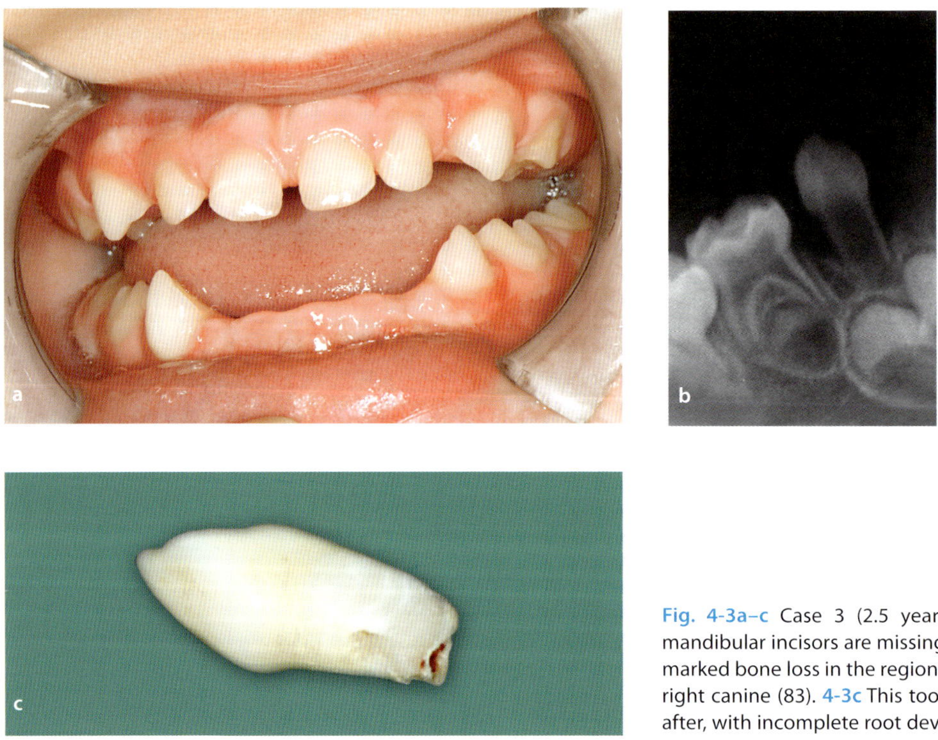

Fig. 4-3a–c Case 3 (2.5 years). 4-3a The four mandibular incisors are missing and 4-3b there is marked bone loss in the region of the mandibular right canine (83). 4-3c This tooth exfoliated soon after, with incomplete root development.

Laboratory Findings
The medical examination revealed pathologically reduced serum ALP activity and raised values of urinary phosphoethanolamine. All other findings were normal. A radiograph of the chest showed normal ribs, but a radiograph of the hand and legs revealed a generally coarse mesh bone pattern in the skeleton. One of the main problems was pain in the legs.

Molecular Biology Screening
Screening for mutation in the *ALPL* gene showed that both parents were carriers of mutations previously described in hypophosphatasia. The mutation from the mother was associated with mild forms of the disease.

CASE 4

History

Medical History
Alexander was the second born of three children. His brother and sister were healthy, and his parents were not related. At 15 years of age, he had nearly normal bone mineral content, but had stopped participating in active sports because of pain in his legs and knees.

Dental History
Alexander was referred to a regional pediatric dentist at 17 months of age for premature loss of the mandibular central incisors (Fig. 4-4). Before he was 2 years old, his maxillary central incisors had also exfoliated (Fig. 4-5). At the age of 15 years he showed high caries activity. The mandibular right first molar (46) had been extracted because of caries. In addition, the maxillary left lateral incisor (22) showed increased mobility.

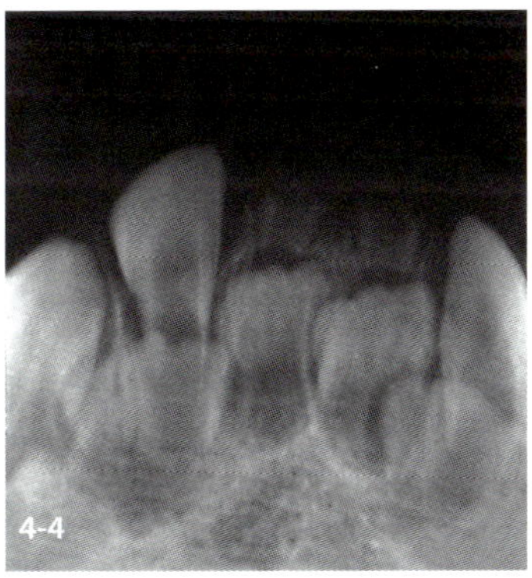

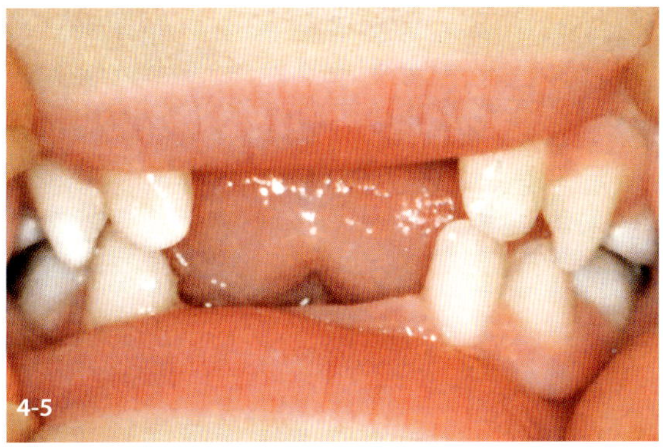

Fig. 4-4 Case 4 (17 months). Apical root fragments of the mandibular central incisors (71, 81) are seen, possibly due to remnants of Hertwig's root sheath.

Fig. 4-5 Case 4 (3 years). There is loss of five primary incisors.

Additional Investigations

Intraoral radiographs of the maxillary and mandibular incisors at 17 months of age revealed findings of hypophosphatasia in the primary teeth (wide pulp chambers in the anterior teeth and early tooth loss in the mandible). Furthermore, as in case 1, the radiographs showed apical root fragments in the region of the early tooth loss (Fig. 4-4). The mandibular central incisors were shed when the patient was 9 months old, probably leaving viable Hertwig's epithelial root sheath in the alveolar socket after exfoliation.

Histologic examination of the maxillary right primary central incisor (51) showed areas with complete absence of cementum and areas with hypomineralized and hypoplastic cementum. Furthermore, there was apical resorption and apical irregular dentin (osteodentin).

A panoramic radiograph at 14 years showed ectopically positioned canines (Fig. 4-6). One year later there was marginal bone loss and cervical resorption on the distal aspect of the maxillary left lateral incisor (22) (Fig. 4-7). Histopathologic examination of the surgically extracted permanent canines also revealed areas with hypoplasia and absence (aplasia) of the cementum.

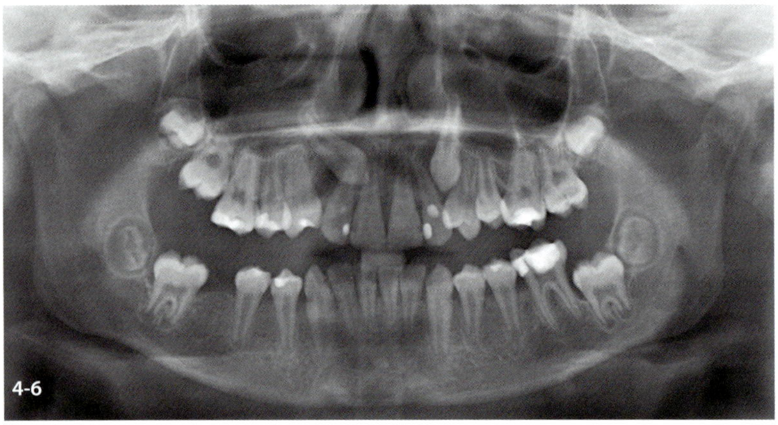

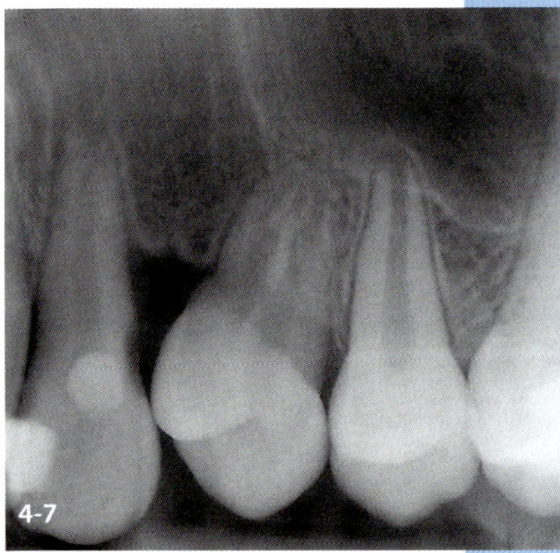

Fig. 4-6 Case 4 (14 years). Ectopically positioned upper canines. The mandibular right first molar (46) has been extracted and he has many restorations.

Fig. 4-7 Case 4 (15 years). Cervical resorption of the maxillary left lateral incisor (22) with loss of bone height. The maxillary left canine (23) was surgically extracted.

Laboratory Findings

The pediatric dentist suspected hypophosphatasia and referred Alexander for additional investigations at the region hospital when he was 20 months of age. Skeletal radiographs showed delayed mineralization. Further examinations at 2½ years of age revealed pathologically reduced serum ALP activity; the level of urinary phosphoethanolamine was six times above the upper end of the normal range. These findings confirmed the clinical diagnosis of hypophosphatasia.

Molecular Biology Screening

A recent screening for mutation in the *ALPL* gene showed that this patient is a compound heterozygote, both parents being carriers of two different, known mutations in the gene. The mutation from the father is associated with mild forms of the disease, and the mutation from the mother with severe forms.

Key Message

All requisitions for screening for the ALPL gene mutations should be sent to Centre Hospitalier de Versailles in France, where it will be catalogued in the worldwide database maintained by Professor Mornet and his group (http://www.sesep.uvsq.fr/Database.html).

TREATMENT AIMS (FOR ALL FOUR CASES)

The aim of dental treatment in such situations is to preserve the forming teeth with suitable preventive programs.

Suspected individuals should also be referred to a pediatrician, who may provide for the necessary examination and additional investigations to confirm the diagnosis and medical follow-up.

Rationale

Premature loss of primary teeth without an underlying systemic disease is rare. There are also conditions other than hypophosphatasia that are associated with tooth loss before the age of 5 years or marked loosening of primary teeth. Aggressive periodontitis, Papillon–Lefèvre syndrome, Coffin–Lowry syndrome, and cyclic neutropenia are some of the conditions which should be considered.[1]

Hypophosphatasia is the systemic disease most often associated with premature tooth loss. This is due to reduced synthesis of the tissue–non-specific ALP enzyme because of mutations in the liver/bone/kidney *ALPL* gene. ALP is particularly active during mineralization and may vary from nearly complete activity to complete loss of activity.[2] Thus the condition manifests as a variety of clinical forms with severity depending on the expressivity or penetration of the gene defect. The disorder may be inherited as an autosomal dominant or recessive trait; the autosomal recessive trait is the most common. The birth prevalence of severe hypophosphatasia is estimated to be 1/100 000, but moderate and mild forms may be much more prevalent.[3]

The clinical manifestations range from stillbirth to pathologic fractures developing only late in adulthood. The earlier the clinical symptoms occur the more serious the disorder usually is. Depending on the age at diagnosis, six forms are described: perinatal (lethal), prenatal benign, infantile, childhood, adult, and odontohypophosphatasia, in which the dental findings are the predominant manifestations of the disease.[3] Hypophosphatasia may be due to different mutations in the *ALPL* gene as described in the four children in this chapter. They all seem to have the childhood type, but with different expressions. The clinical manifestations for cases 1 and 4 may so far also fit the odontohypophosphatasia type.

Key Messages

Hypophosphatasia should be considered in any patient with a history of early unexplained loss of teeth or abnormal loss of teeth.

If hypophosphatasia is considered, levels of phosphoethanolamine in the urine and ALP in serum should be measured. Pathologically reduced levels of serum ALP and raised levels of phosphoethanolamine in urine are reliable diagnostic indicators.

Skeletal pain can cause physical impairment.

TREATMENT

General issues

There is no established or curative treatment for hypophosphatasia, but the correct diagnosis helps to avoid the use of therapies for other diseases with inadequate skeletal mineralization. Thus the medical treatment has so far, in the present cases, been recommendation of symptomatic anti-inflammatory treatment with non-steroidal anti-inflammatory drugs (NSAIDs) to relieve pain from joints and muscles. NSAIDs have been shown to considerably improve pain-associated physical impairment and pain in the lower limbs without evident fractures; the pain may be due to elevated levels of prostaglandins.[4] Physiotherapy is also a part of the medical treatment. Furthermore, regular medical follow-up and radiographic examinations are required to monitor bone density. All the four children in this chapter were classified as ASA II.

For each patient, an oral hygiene program has been designed, aiming to preserve the remaining periodontium. Information and instruction in dental hygiene is given and they have regular visits to the dental clinic for professional cleaning.

Two of the children have permanent teeth which so far show normal bone height, except the maxillary lateral incisors in case 4 following the removal of his upper canines. With regard to case 1, a thorough discussion has been performed with an orthodontist. It was decided to extract just the maxillary right first premolar (14) to avoid orthodontic treatment. There is a lack of literature supporting orthodontic treatment in hypophosphatasia patients. In case 1, longer use of the partial denture might have prevented the migration of teeth. Both she, and, in particular, case 4 have many restorations in their permanent teeth, which indicates high caries activity.

Key Messages

Wide pulp chambers should be taken into consideration during cavity preparation.

An orthodontist should be consulted at an early age as it is not clear whether orthodontic tooth movement can be recommended due to the underlying cementum deficiency in patients with hypophosphatasia.

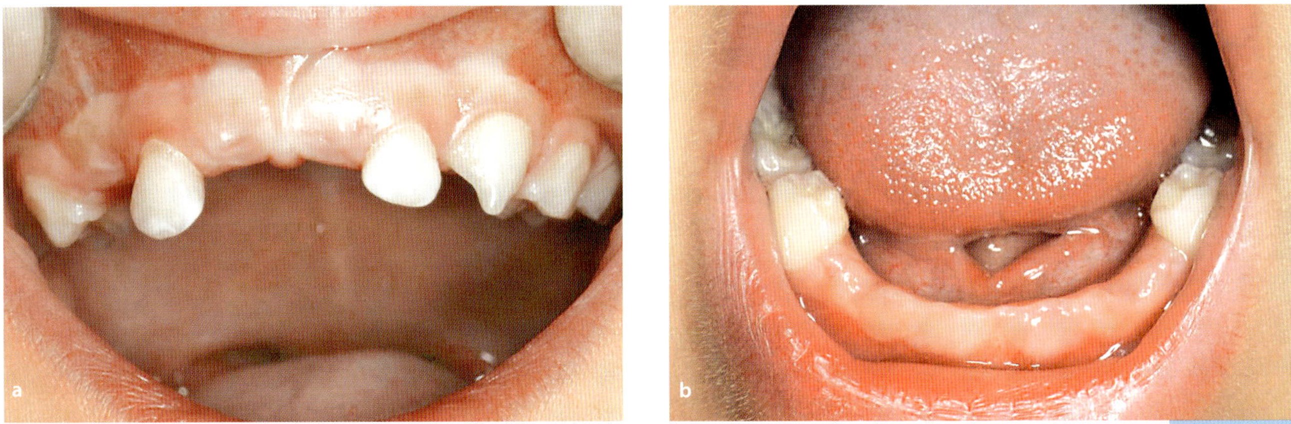

Fig. 4-8a,b Case 1 (2.5 years). Nine primary teeth have been lost. Both the maxillary lateral incisors (52 and 62) have small opacities.

Case 1

Agnes was followed up by her local dentist with intermittent consultations at the department of pediatric dentistry. At 32 months of age, all the mandibular anterior teeth were exfoliated; in the maxilla, the right central incisor and canine and the left central incisor (51, 53, 61) were lost (Figs 4-8a, 4-8b). By the age of 4 years, no more teeth were shed, but all the remaining teeth, except the second primary molars, were mobile. The patient experienced no problem with eating or talking, and she had no pain, but other children commented on her missing teeth.

At the age of 5 years, the maxillary right lateral incisor (52) was also shed, and soon after the maxillary left first primary molar (64) as well. She was conscious about her lack of teeth and she was fitted with partial dentures in the upper and lower jaws. However, the upper denture was lost after half a year, and when she began attending school, she accepted her situation after observing other children with exfoliated teeth.

At present, the patient is 10½ years old and in the late mixed dentition. There is crowding in the maxilla and insufficient space, in particular for the right canine, because of the premature tooth loss and tooth migration (Figs 4-9a, 4-9b). Serial extractions might have been performed, but the family had moved several times and regular follow-up had been difficult. The maxillary right first premolar will be extracted in the near future to allow the canine to erupt.

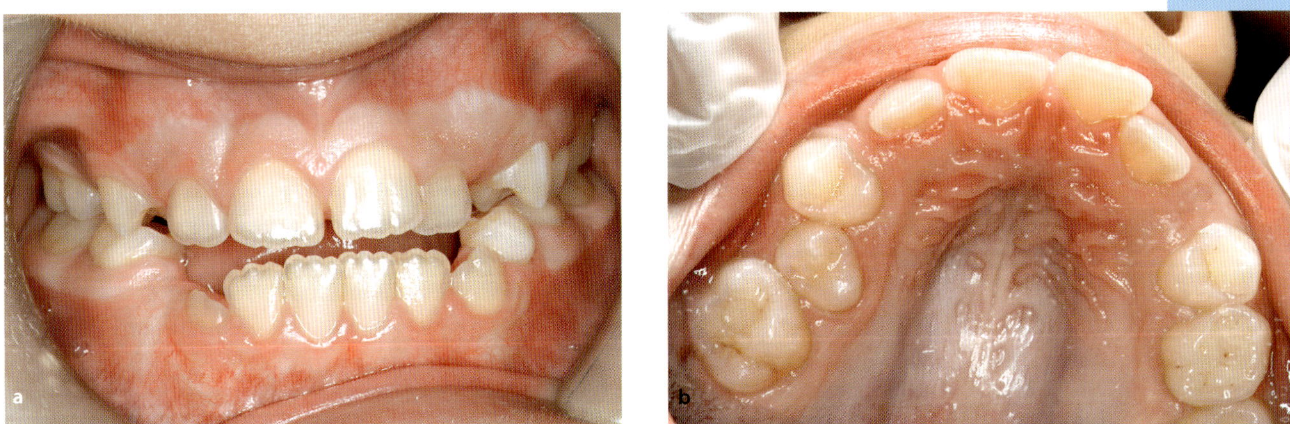

Fig. 4-9a,b Case 1 (10.5 years). Mixed dentition, distal occlusion with crowding in the maxilla.

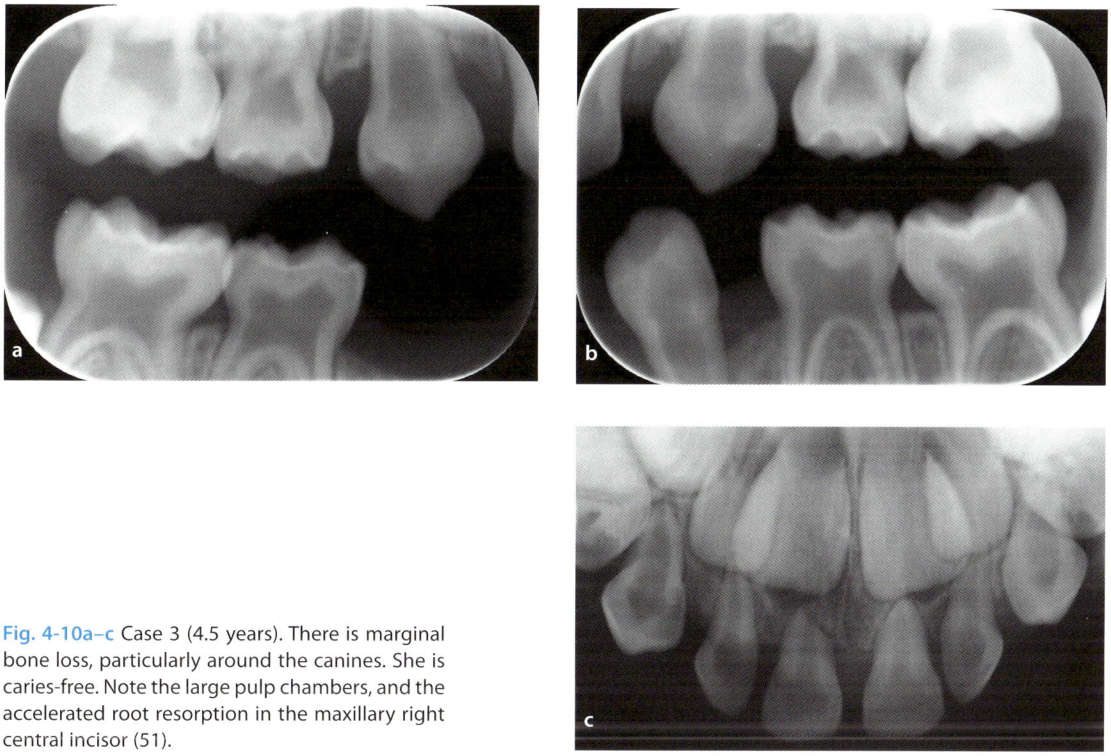

Fig. 4-10a–c Case 3 (4.5 years). There is marginal bone loss, particularly around the canines. She is caries-free. Note the large pulp chambers, and the accelerated root resorption in the maxillary right central incisor (51).

Case 2

Carious lesions in the mandibular primary second molars (75, 85) were treated by the local dentist. The oral hygienist had arranged regular recall visits, but the family had moved and follow-up was complicated.

A recent medical follow-up revealed that the siblings were stiff legged, Peter more than his sister (see case 1). He had pain in his feet and legs, and he is unable to run and jump as much as other children. He has regular physiotherapy as well as swimming-pool training.

NSAIDs were tried, but with no evident effect. Skeleton radiographs show slight sclerosis, common for the disorder.

Case 3

Stephanie is being followed up by her local dentist. Her oral hygiene is good and there is no sign of carious lesions (Figs 4-10a, 4-10b). At the age of 4 she injured her maxillary right primary central incisor (51) and subsequent accelerated root resorption has been observed (Fig. 4-10c).

Stephanie used NSAIDs (ibuprofen mixture) regularly from 3 to 4 years of age with good clinical effect reducing pain and improving motor functions. For the time being the medication is only used at need. She has physiotherapy every week.

Case 4

Alexander had high caries activity despite thorough and regular follow-up. He accumulated plaque easily. The maxillary right first molar (16) had been extracted when he was 13 years old. At the age of 15 years none of the permanent teeth were mobile except for the maxillary left lateral incisor (22). Following surgical removal of the non-erupted, ectopically positioned upper canines, he has all his permanent teeth, except the mandibular right first molar (46). The decision to remove the canines instead of having orthodontic treatment was made because of the uncertainty concerning the prognosis of the teeth after orthodontic tooth movement. The resorption defect in the maxillary left lateral incisor (22) has been treated by removal of granulation tissue and curettage during a flap operation. The defect was smaller than suspected and removal of infected/inflamed tissue around the involved tooth promoted healing of the periodontal tissue and reduced the pocket depth.

DISCUSSION

If primary teeth are lost before the normal time of shedding without an obvious reason, the child should be referred for further consideration. A considerable challenge is to preserve as many teeth as possible. A common feature in patients with hypophosphatasia is involvement of the cementum, which is affected to a greater or lesser extent (aplasia and hypoplasia, respectively). Moreover, reduced alveolar bone height without gingival inflammation and enlarged pulp chambers are also common findings.[5,6] These defects have more often been described in the primary teeth, but similar changes have also been found in the permanent dentition.[7,8] Apical areas of "osteodentin" were observed in case 4, also described previously.[7]

The irregular cementum affects the periodontal attachment, and may facilitate the down growth of bacteria along the root surface, thus accelerating tooth loss. In case 4, cervical root resorption of the maxillary left lateral incisor (22) has been diagnosed. Roots with deficient cementum are more prone to resorption, and in this case it might have been caused by pressure from neighboring teeth. Thus, children with hypophosphatasia are at risk of developing oral complications during adolescence and adult life, which should be taken into consideration by the dentist when planning preventive strategies and treatment.

A study comparing primary teeth with hypophosphatasia with matched controls[9] did not find any difference in the mineral content of the dentin, but both acellular and cellular cement formation was affected. The authors concluded that different regulatory mechanisms operate for mineralization in these two tissues. However, disturbed mineralization of coronal dentin in permanent teeth has been reported.[8] Regarding enamel mineralization, there is limited information, but cases with enamel hypoplasia[6] and cases where caries is the main problem in the permanent dentition[10] have been reported.

In two of the present cases (cases 1 and 4) apical root fragments were observed in the absence of previous trauma history. This may be a result of continued root development from remnants of viable Hertwig's epithelial root sheath in the alveolar socket after the early tooth exfoliation.

It may seem that the activity of the biochemical defect is greatest in the early years of life as the dental involvement is greatest in the first erupted primary teeth and more seldom affects the permanent teeth. Patients with adult hypophosphatasia or odontohypophosphatasia are believed to have a normal lifespan.[3]

REFERENCES

1. Hartsfield JK. Premature exfoliation of teeth in childhood and adolescence. Adv Pediatr 1994;41:453–470.
2. Whyte MP. Hypophosphatasia and the role of alkaline phosphatase in skeletal mineralization. Endocr Rev 1994;15:439–461.
3. Mornet E. Hypophosphatasia. Orphanet J Rare Dis 2007;2:40.
4. Girschick HJ, Schneider P, Haubitz I, Hiort O, Collmann H, Beer M, et al. Effective NSAID treatment indicates that hyperprostaglandinism is affecting the clinical severity of childhood hypophosphatasia. Orphanet J Rare Dis 2006;1:24.
5. Lundgren T, Westphal O, Bolme P, Modèer T, Norèn JG. Retrospective study of children with hypophosphatasia with reference to dental changes. Scand J Dent Res 1991;99:357–364.
6. Ritchie GM. Hypophosphatasia. A metabolic disease with important dental manifestations. Arch Dis Child 1964;39:584–590.
7. El-Labban NG, Lee KW, Rule D. Permanent teeth in hypophosphatasia: light and electron microscopic study. J Oral Pathol Med 1991;20:352–360.
8. Olsson A, Matsson L, Blomquist HK, Larsson A, Sjödin B. Hypophosphatasia affecting the permanent dentition. J Oral Pathol Med 1996;25:343–347.
9. van den Bos T, Handoko G, Niehof A, Ryan LM, Coburn SP, Whyte MP, et al. Cementum and dentin in hypophosphatasia. J Dent Res 2005;84:1021–1025.
10. Lepe X, Rothwell BR, Banich S, Page RC. Absence of adult dental anomalies in familial hypophosphatasia. J Periodontal Res 1997;32:375–380.

5

Non-operative Management of Dental Caries in the Primary Dentition

Dafydd Evans
Nicola Innes

Key words: carious primary teeth, fluoride varnish, prevention, toothbrushing

Age category: 4–7 years

Definition
Non-operative management of dental caries in the primary dentition is an alternative to the surgical approach of caries excision followed by conventional fillings. It is a prevention-alone approach, based on biologic management of the plaque biofilm. This may slow or arrest dental caries sufficiently for the primary tooth to exfoliate without causing pain or dental infection.

Despite a decline in caries prevalence over the past few decades, the World Health Organization (WHO) report[1] in 2003 stated "Dental caries is still a major oral health problem in most industrialised countries, affecting sixty to ninety percent of schoolchildren". In Scotland in 2006, 46% of 5-year-old children had clinically obvious dental caries.[2] Progressive dental caries can lead to pain and dental infection unless it is managed. Traditional forms of managing the disease involve removing infected tooth tissue with rotary instruments, and then restoring the tooth with a plastic filling material or a preformed metal crown. Local anesthesia is usually used to allow the procedure to be carried out without the child experiencing pain. However, it can be difficult for young children to accept this treatment, especially at the beginning of their dental experiences.

THE PROBLEM

Paul (aged 5 years) was referred by his general dental practitioner to the children's department at Dundee Dental Hospital for dental extractions under general anesthesia. On examination, he was found to have a complete primary dentition, with every tooth affected by dental caries. The carious lesions were advanced in many of the teeth, with several being unrestorable. Paul's mother did not want his care to involve the use of general anesthesia, and wished to avoid extractions. He was not experiencing pain in any teeth, and there were no clinical signs or symptoms of dental infection (such as pain, swelling or alveolar inflammation). It was, therefore, decided to manage his dental disease with an intensive prevention program, to allow his confidence to build to a level where he would be happy to accept invasive treatment.

CASE DESCRIPTION

History

Medical History
ASA I. Paul was fit and well. He had very mild eczema, but otherwise there was no contributory medical history.

Dental History
Paul had only recently attended a general dental practitioner, who had referred him to Dundee Dental Hospital and School for dental extractions under general anesthesia, as he felt that Paul's dental

caries was too extensive for him to manage. Paul's mother reported that he had never complained of any dental pain, nor had there been any facial swellings, and that he had no difficulty eating his food.

Examination

On examination, all 20 primary teeth were found to be present, and all were affected by dental caries (Figs 5-1a to 5-1c). Careful examination of the soft tissues showed no signs of dental infection, such as a sinus from a dental abscess. A pulp polyp was present on the mandibular right primary second molar (85). It was decided that radiographic information would not alter the provisional treatment plan, so radiographs were not taken at this time.

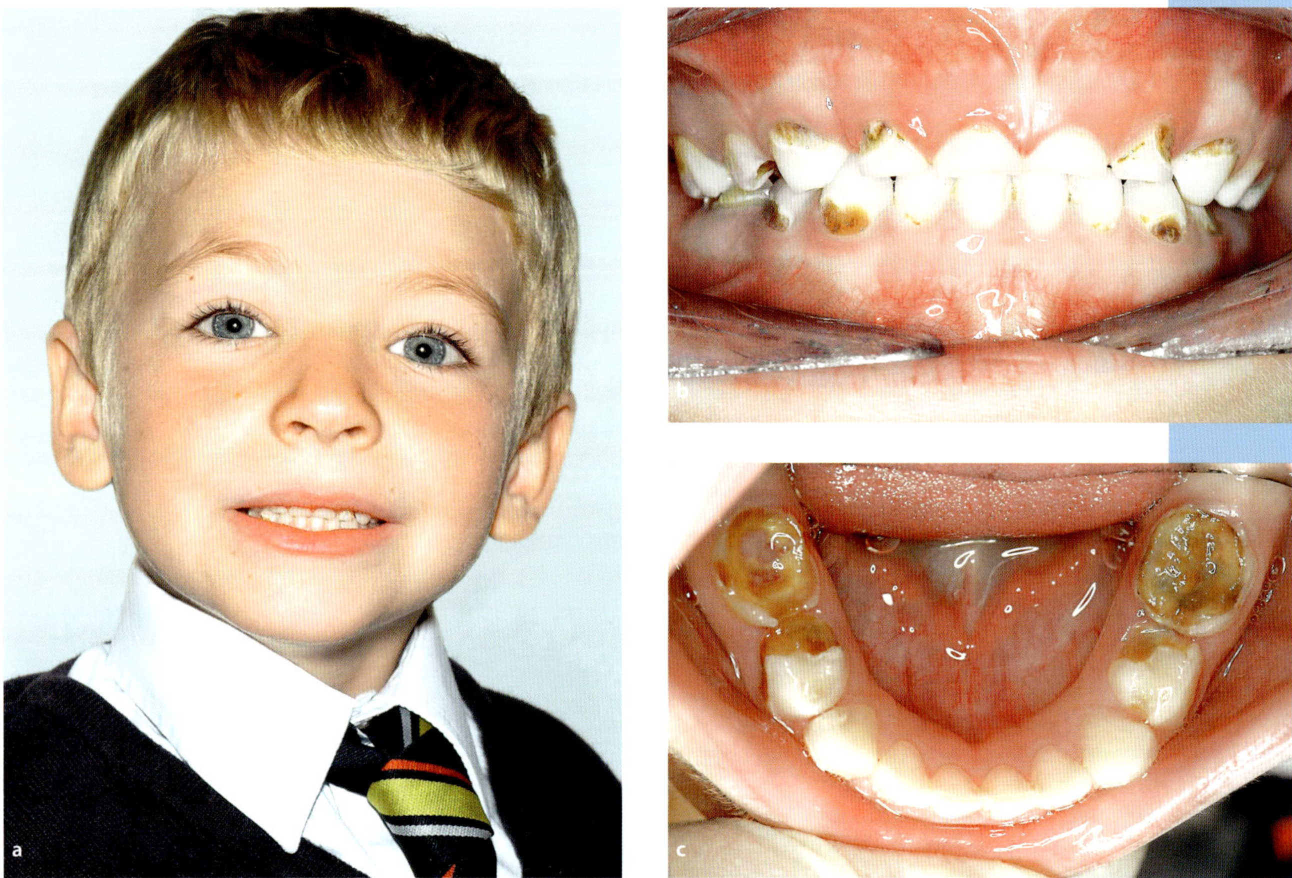

Fig. 5-1a–c Initial assessment (age 5 years 6 months).

TREATMENT AIMS

Avoid surgical management of the dental caries until the patient's confidence had built up to the level where he would accept treatment with local anesthesia.

Prevent the dental caries from causing any pain or dental infection until that stage was reached, using an intensive caries preventive program.

TREATMENT PLAN

Provisional Treatment Plan

An intensive caries preventive program, with:

- "hands-on" toothbrushing instruction with the patient's mother, which involved disclosing plaque and a combination of observing her toothbrushing technique and offering advice to both her and the patient on how the effectiveness of brushing could be maximized

- general toothbrushing advice, following national guidelines[3] (adult toothpaste with ≥1000 ppm fluoride; twice daily brushing; spitting out, but not rinsing, after brushing)
- home use of a calcium phosphate based remineralization system[4] (Tooth Mousse™ GC)
- professionally applied fluoride varnish (Duraphat™, Colgate) three times per year
- investigation of diet habits, and discussion and advice on reducing the frequency of cariogenic attacks.

Definitive Treatment Plan

As long as the intensive preventive program was successful in keeping Paul free from pain and dental Infection, this was to continue. However, if there was continued tooth breakdown, or if pain or dental infection developed, this was to be managed with restorations, pulp therapy or extraction, if Paul would allow it. If he was too anxious to accept this treatment, then the possible use of general anesthesia for extractions was to be renegotiated with his mother.

Rationale

There were several factors which made following a traditional approach to managing our patient's caries problematic. These included: his young age, the number of teeth affected, the extent of the disease in many of the teeth, his mother's wish to avoid the use of general anesthesia, and his limited experience of dental treatment. As the history and clinical examination indicated that he did not have any pain or dental infection, a prevention-alone approach was adopted, which included brushing instruction, diet advice, fluoride varnish and Tooth Mousse. It was anticipated that by avoiding highly invasive treatments such as extractions and pulp therapy at initial appointments, Paul's perceptions of dental treatment would be positive. This would allow him time to acclimatize to the dental environment and this, together with him becoming older, would increase his ability to accept the use of local anesthetic injections. The key factors in the approach were:

- managing the carious lesions biologically (rather than surgically), by disrupting and removing the plaque biofilm on the surface of the lesions through effective, parent-led toothbrushing
- ensuring that the mother understood and accepted that responsibility for the success of the management program lay with her and not with the dental practitioner.

TREATMENT AND FOLLOW-UP

Treatment

Treatment was based on intensive, hands-on toothbrushing instruction with Paul and his mother. In addition, Paul's diet was investigated through a diet diary, which was discussed with him and his mother, and changes suggested. Paul was given Tooth Mousse to use at home, and fluoride varnish was also applied three times a year. He and his mother were advised that if Paul experienced pain at any time, then he was to return immediately for assessment.

Follow-up

3 months (Figs 5-2a to 5-2d)

At the 3-month review, Paul reported no pain, and his plaque control was seen to have improved. Fluoride varnish was applied. Dietary habits and changes were discussed again, with key messages reinforced.

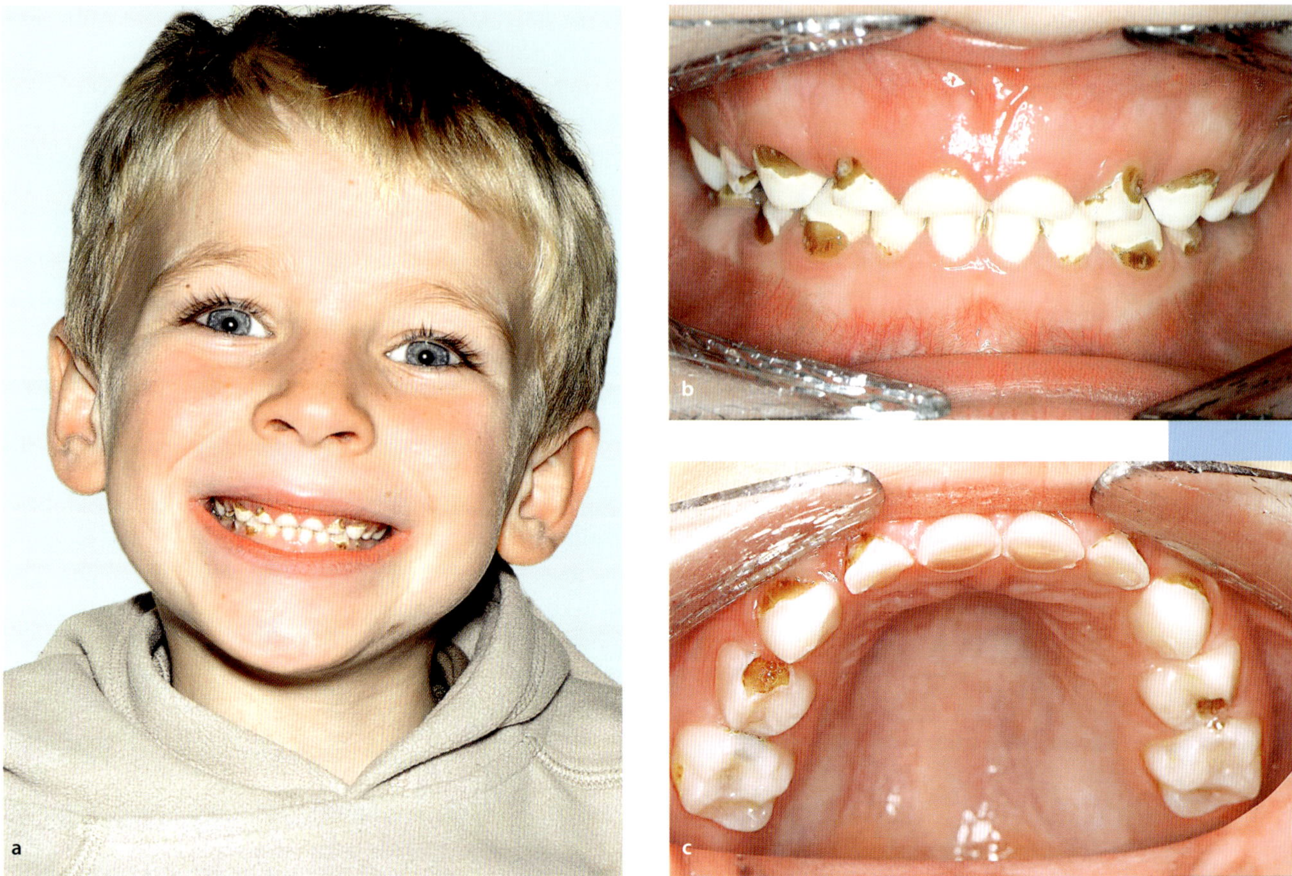

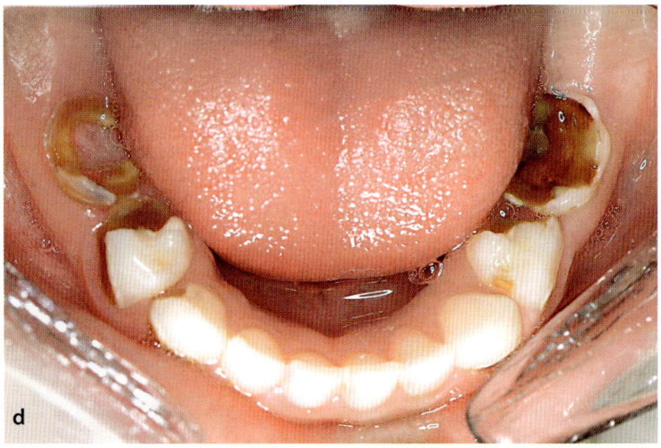

Fig. 5-2a–d Post assessment – 3 months (age $5\frac{3}{4}$ years).

8 months (Figs 5-3a to 5-3c)

At the 8-month review, again there was no report of any problems, and many of the carious lesions were noted to have changed colour and darkened. The pulp polyp at the mandibular right primary second molar (85) was now confluent with the lingual gingival margin, and the surface of the mandibular left primary second molar (75) was becoming harder.

14 months (Figs 5-4a to 5-4c)

At the 14-month review, most of the carious lesions were darker in colour, and there were no signs or symptoms of dental infection. The lower first permanent molars were erupting, and as the patient was considered to be high caries risk, these were sealed with glass-ionomer cement (Fuji VII™, GC) while partially erupted, to keep them caries-free until it was possible to place resin sealants.

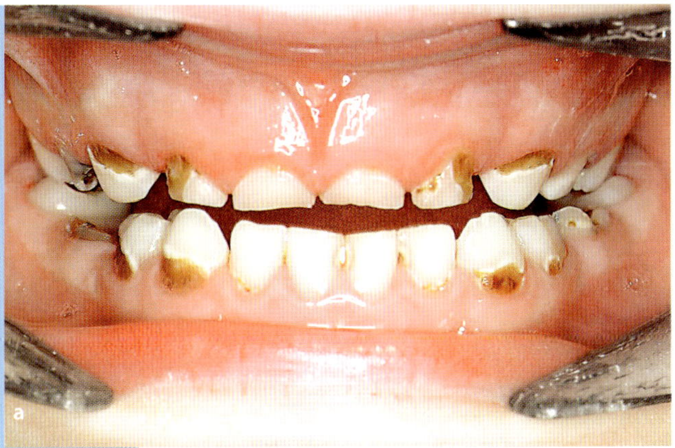

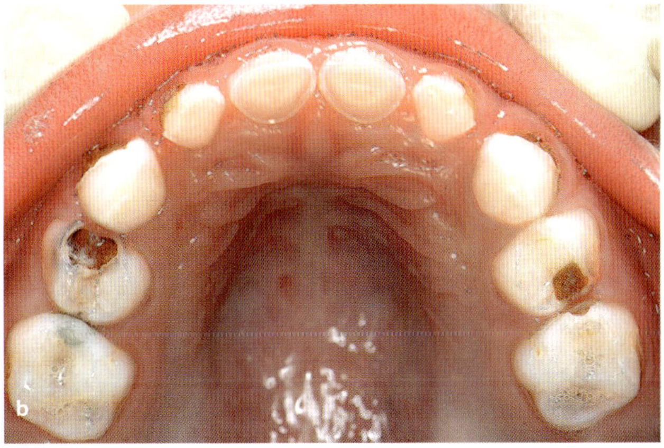

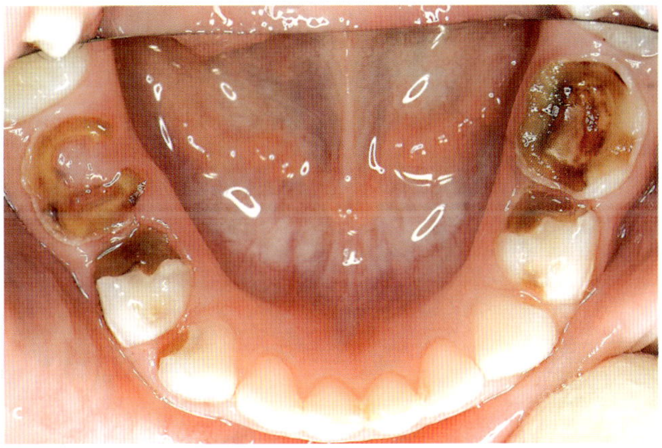

Fig. 5-3a–c Post assessment – 8 months (age 6 years).

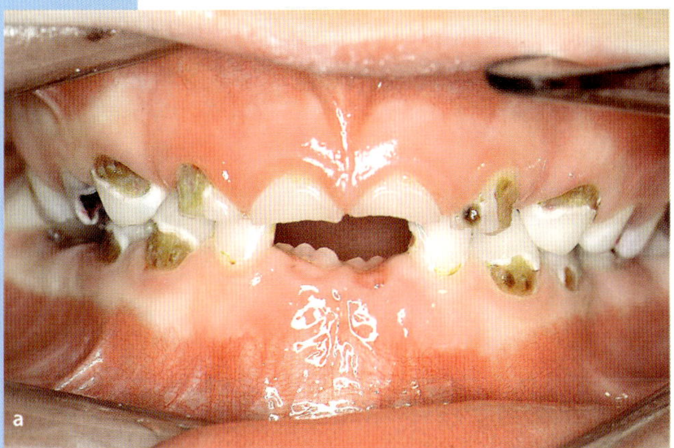

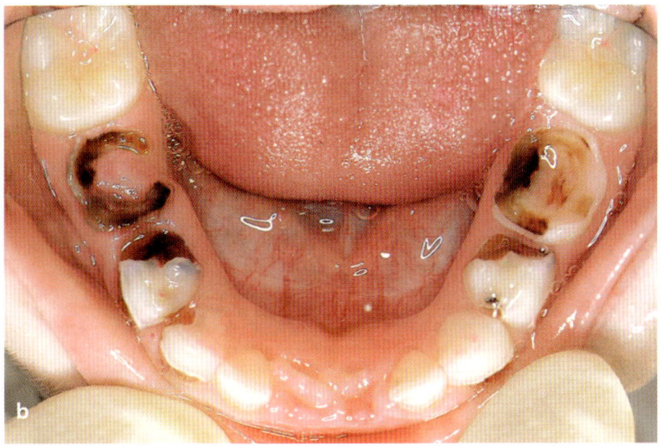

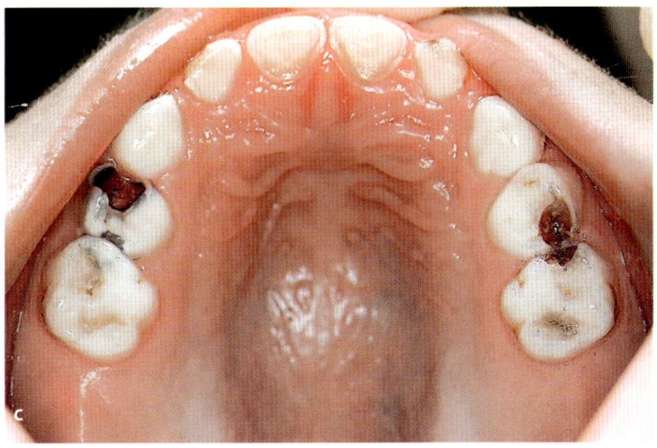

Fig. 5-4a–c Post assessment – 14 months (age 6½ years).

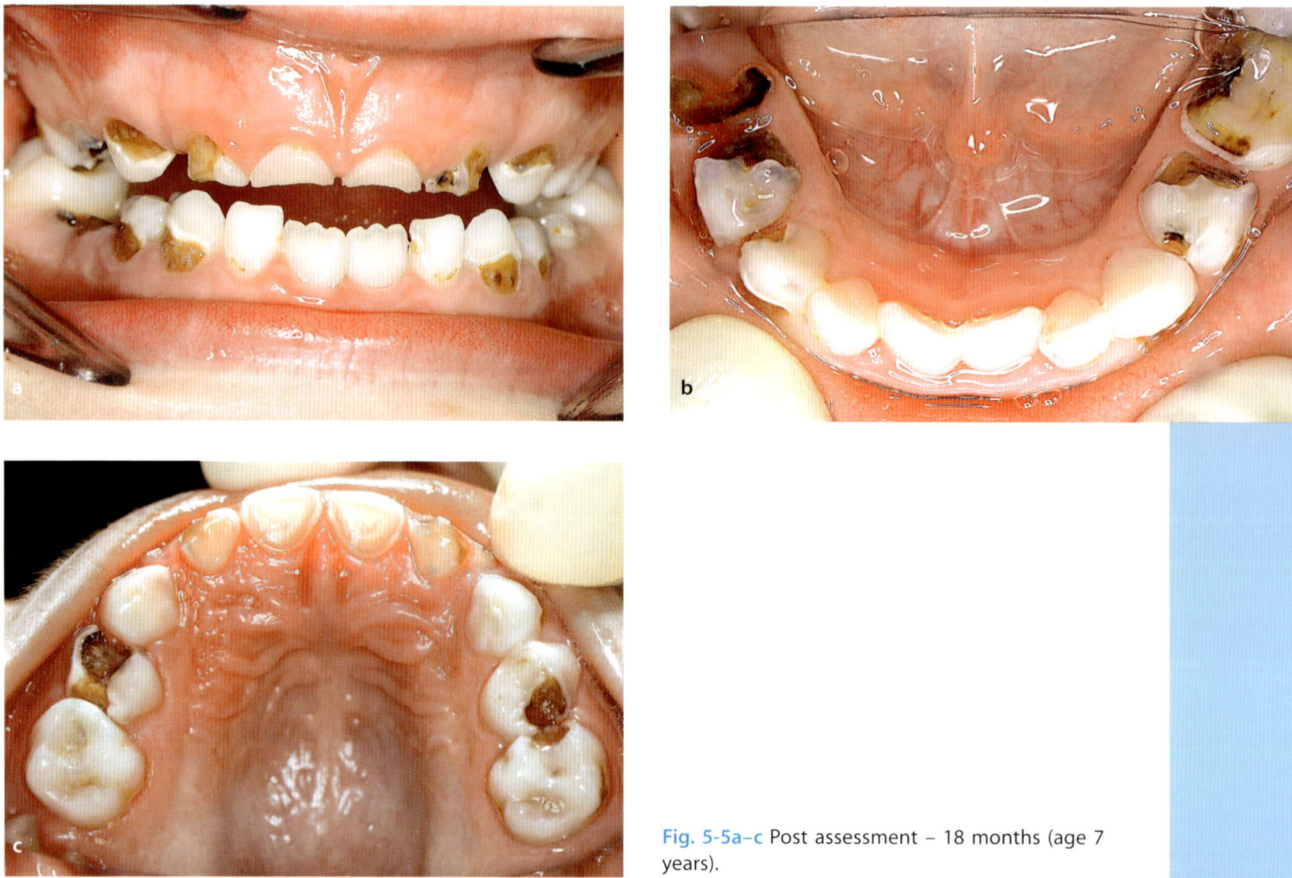

Fig. 5-5a–c Post assessment – 18 months (age 7 years).

18 months (Figs 5-5a to 5-5c)

At the 18-month review, history and clinical examination indicated that the prevention-alone approach had been successful in preventing pain and dental infection. Carious lesions in the mandibular quadrants appeared clinically to be arresting, although some caries progression was noted in the maxillary molars. Toothbrushing was emphasized, as plaque control was more effective in the mandibular than the maxillary arch, as is apparent from Figure 5-5.

24 months (Figs 5-6a to 5-6d)

A review 2 years after the initial assessment found no signs of dental infection, and all four permanent molars fully erupted. Further resorption of the mandibular right primary second molar (85) had occurred, and the surface of the mandibular left primary second molar (75) was now polished in appearance. Some caries progression in the maxillary molars was noted, where again there was a problem with adequate plaque control. Toothbrushing advice was reinforced.

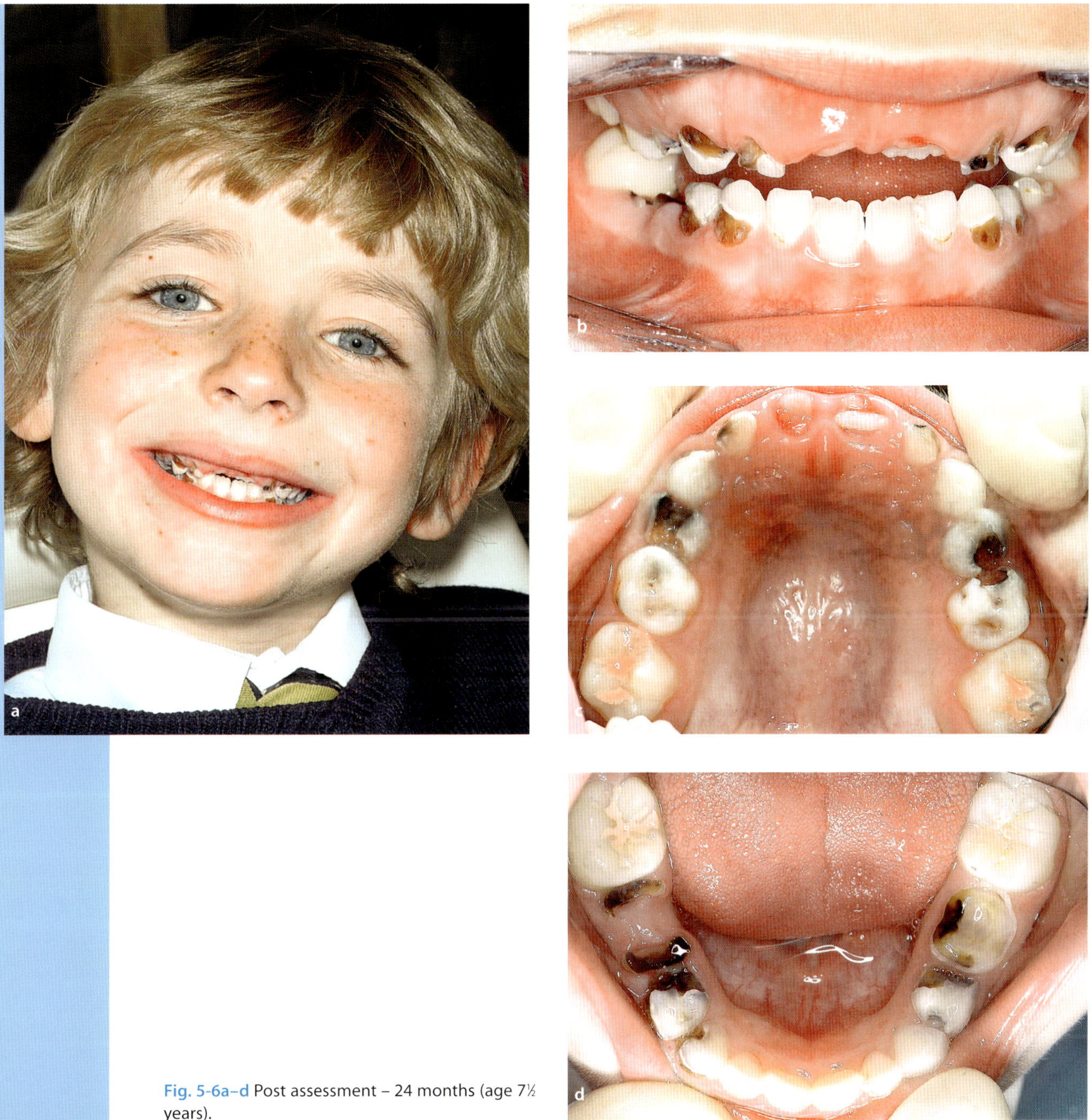

Fig. 5-6a–d Post assessment – 24 months (age 7½ years).

30 months (Figs 5-7a to 5-7e)

Two and a half years after the initial assessment, radiographs were taken to screen for caries in the permanent molars, and these, along with clinical examination, revealed no signs of dental infection. Plaque control, particularly in the maxillary arch, remained problematic, and possibly as a consequence of this, caries progression did not seem to have been slowed to the same extent as in the mandibular arch. The mandibular right primary second molar (85) was now almost completely resorbed, and the surface of the mandibular left primary second molar (75) appeared polished and smooth, with the pulp canal obliteration visible radiographically, indicating it was vital. The glass-ionomer sealants on the permanent molars were replaced with transparent resin sealants.

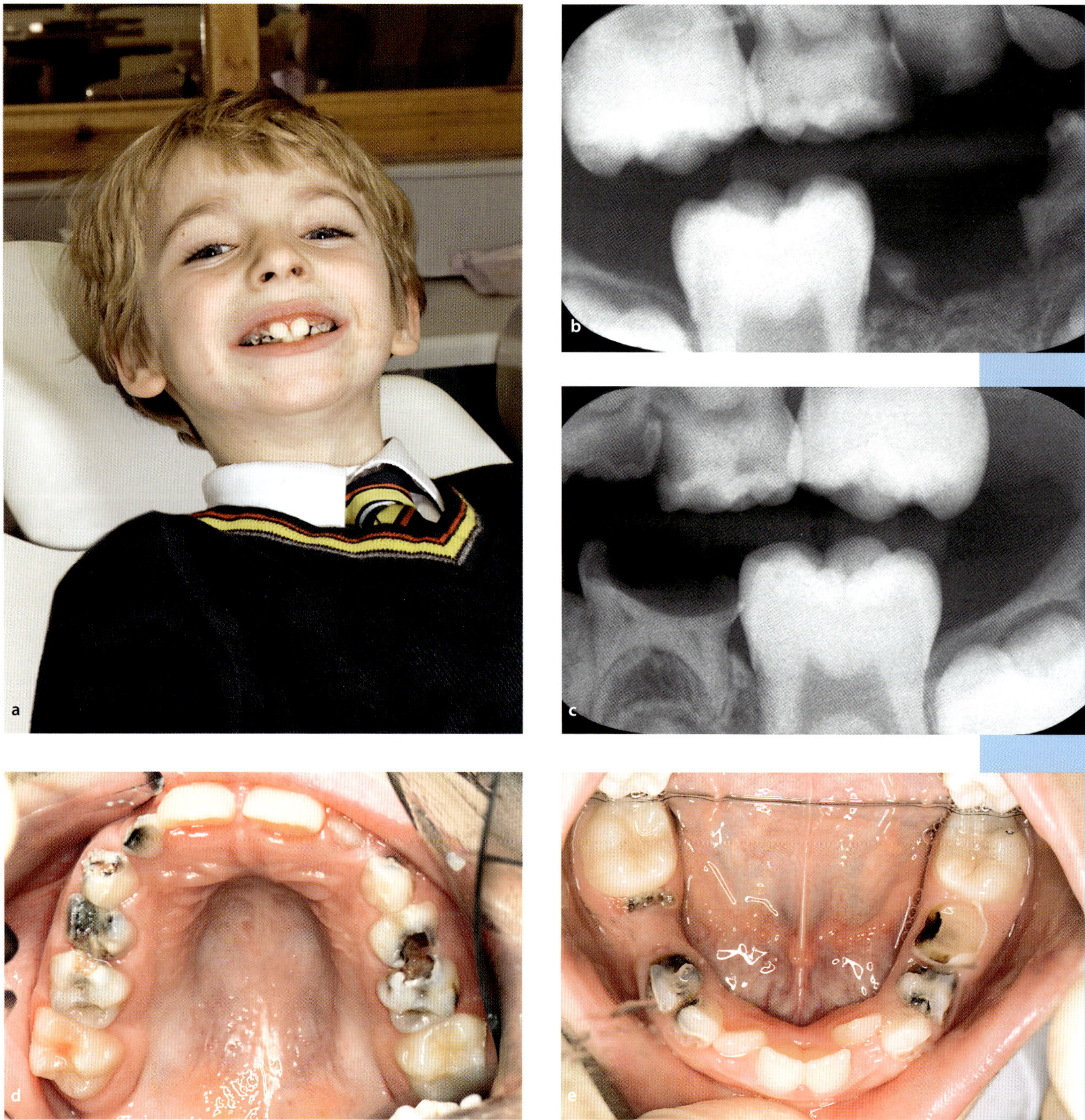

Fig. 5-7a–e Post assessment – 30 months (age 8 years).

36 months (Figs 5-8a to 5-8c)

At latest recall, 3 years after initial assessment, Paul continued to be free from pain and there were no signs or symptoms of dental infection. In view of continued difficulty with plaque control in the maxillary arch (compare with the mandibular arch in Fig. 5-8), and continued caries progression in the maxillary molars, the decision was taken to restore the maxillary primary second molars (55, 65) with preformed metal crowns, using an indirect pulp cap technique.[5] Now that the patient was happy to sit in the dental chair, it was not anticipated that he would have any difficulty accepting this treatment.

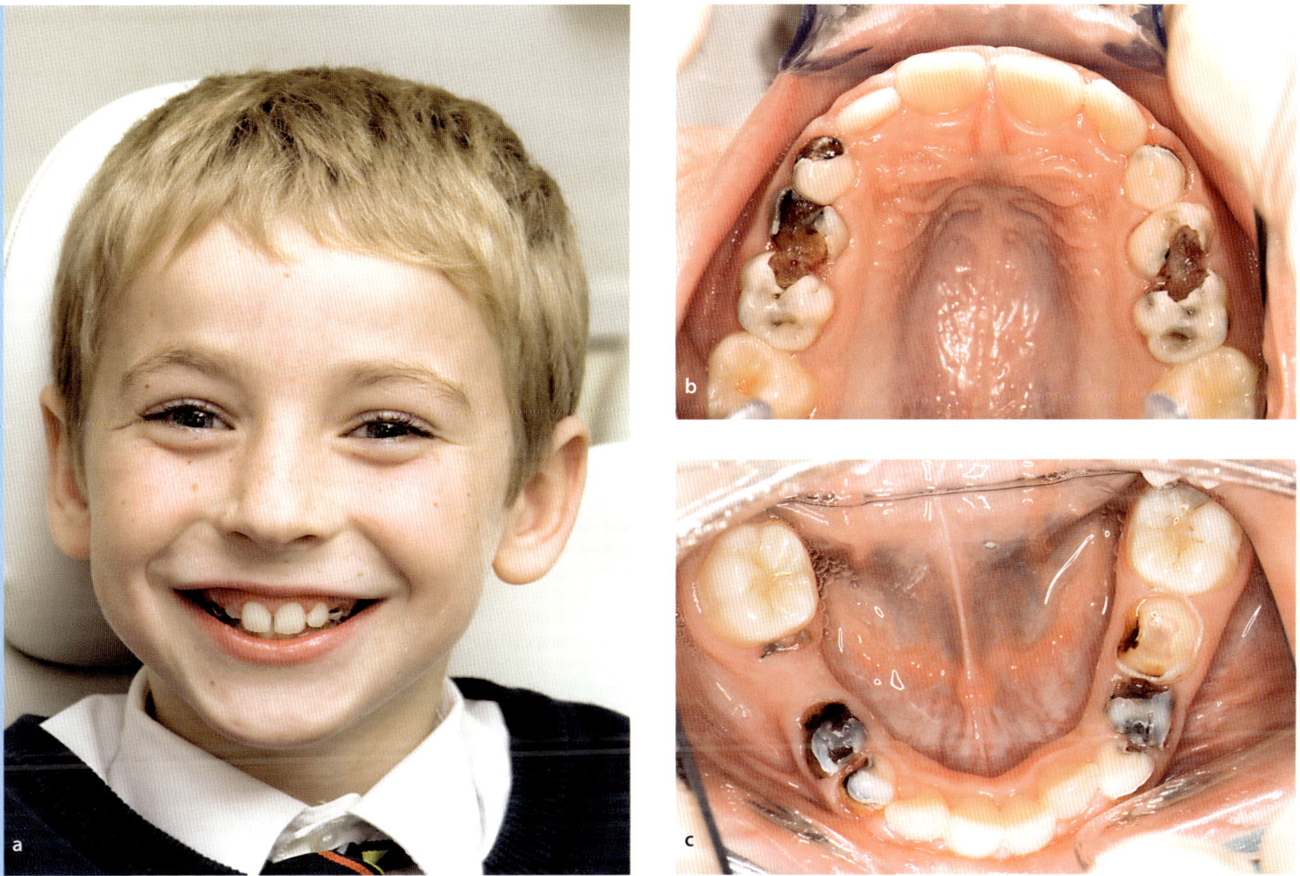

Fig. 5-8a–c Post assessment – 36 months (age 8½ years).

> ***Key Message***
> *A prevention-alone strategy may be appropriate for managing cleansable carious lesions in the primary dentition, if avoidance of pain, dental infection, and treatment-induced anxiety is the principal goal of dental care.*

DISCUSSION

Current best practice for managing carious primary teeth, as defined by guidance from specialist societies, is to remove infected carious tooth tissue, and place a filling.[6] This can be challenging both for the child and the dental practitioner, and the majority of carious primary teeth in young children remain unrestored.[3] As a consequence, pain and dental infection are part of everyday life for many children in the UK.[7] There is, however, growing evidence that the progress of carious lesions can be slowed, or even arrested, by a biologic approach, rather than relying on complete surgical excision.[8,9]

> ***Key Message***
> *The premise of the biologic approach is that the carious process is driven by the plaque biofilm on the surface of a lesion, and that the biofilm is only actively cariogenic under specific environmental conditions, making it vulnerable to manipulation of that environment.[10] Essentially, on disruption of the environment of the plaque biofilm, lesion progression should slow down or even arrest.*

Evidence of this is visible in daily clinical practice involving children, where arrested white spot lesions on the mesial surface of first permanent molars are commonly seen following loss of the second primary molar. For our patient, a prevention-alone approach has kept him free from pain and dental infection for 3 years, and without risk of acquiring treatment-induced anxiety through trying to provide fillings or extractions before he was able to accept them.

It is interesting to note the gradual resorption of the mandibular right primary second molar (85) over the 3 years of observation, without causing pain or dental infection; this supports the view of many clinicians that primary molars with pulp polyps can simply be kept under observation, unless symptomatic. More extraordinary is the change of the surface of the mandibular left primary second molar (75) from soft, brown dental caries to the hard, polished surface seen after 3 years, with every indication that the dental pulp had either survived, or possibly revascularized once the bacterial ingress from the surface plaque biofilm had been reduced by toothbrushing, or possibly due to the other preventive measures. It is interesting to speculate that the apparently greater success of the prevention-alone approach in the mandibular arch compared with the maxillary arch (where caries progression continued to some extent, although slowly) was due to the cleansability of the initial lesions, which were more open.

It is not possible to determine the relative contribution of the various components of our patient's preventive program in keeping him free from pain and dental infection. It is likely, however, that a key part was played, at least initially, by his mother in maintaining meticulous plaque control over the surface of the carious lesions. A prevention-alone approach relies heavily on the child's parent for its success, and this approach may not be successful where parental motivation is poor, or when the child takes over responsibility for toothbrushing from their parent, as they get older.

REFERENCES

1 The World Oral Health Report 2003 website. Available at: www.who.int/oral_health/media/en/orh_report03_en.pdf. Accessed 13 March 2009.

2 National Dental Inspection Programme of Scotland: Report of the 2006 Survey of P1 Children website. Available at: www.scottishdental.org/?record=71. Accessed 13 March 2009.

3 Scottish Intercollegiate Guidelines Network website. Prevention and Management of Decay in the Pre-school Child: SIGN Guideline 83, 2005. Available at: www.sign.ac.uk/pdf/sign83.pdf. Accessed 13 March 2009.

4 Reynolds EC. Calcium phosphate-based remineralization systems: Scientific evidence? Aust Dent J 2008;53:268–273.

5 Coll JA. Indirect pulp capping and primary teeth: is the primary tooth pulpotomy out of date? J Endodont 2008;34(7 suppl.):S34–S39.

6 Fayle SA, Welbury RR, Roberts JF. British Society of Paediatric Dentistry: a policy document on management of caries in the primary dentition. Int J Paediatr Dent 2001;11:153–157.

7 Shepherd MA, Nadanovsky P, Sheiham A. The prevalence and impact of dental pain in 8-year-old school children in Harrow, England. Br Dent J 1999;187:38–41.

8 Ricketts DN, Kidd EA, Innes N, Clarkson J. Complete or ultraconservative removal of decayed tissue in unfilled teeth. Cochrane Database Syst Rev. 2006;(3):CD003808.

9 Innes NPT, Evans DJP, Stirrups DR. The Hall Technique: a randomized controlled clinical trial of a novel method of managing carious primary molars in general dental practice; acceptability of the technique and outcomes at 23 months. BMC Oral Health 2007;7:18.

10 Marsh PD. Dental plaque as a microbial biofilm. Caries Res 2004;38:204–211.

6

Role of the Pediatric Dentist in Hypodontia

Julie Caroline Mitchell
Marie Therese Hosey

Key words: hypodontia, congenitally missing teeth, resin-retained bridges

Age category: 12–18 years

Definition
Hypodontia is the congenital absence of the normal complement of teeth. The most frequently missing teeth are the second premolars, upper laterals, and third molars. The prevalence of hypodontia has been reported to be 3.5–6.5%, with an even higher percentage in Scandinavian children. It is associated with microdontia and other anomalies such as conical shaped teeth, retained primary teeth, and reduced alveolar development.[1,2]

The management of hypodontia is multidisciplinary with orthodontic, restorative, and surgical specialties all involved in the pediatric dentistry case management.[3] Children with congenitally missing teeth are most commonly referred in the mixed dentition period since this is when the disorder is most often recognized, usually because of retention of primary teeth or due to poor esthetics. However, a child might be concerned about their appearance before this age and so it is important for the pediatric dentist not only to recognize but also to provide intermediate management whenever required.[4]

THE PROBLEM

A 14-year-old African Caribbean girl was referred by her dentist for bilateral spaces in the maxillary incisor area. She had congenitally missing maxillary lateral incisors (12, 22). She had completed orthodontic fixed appliance therapy to open up the lateral incisor spaces. The general dentist was querying the possibility of implants. She was wearing a removable retainer but there was insufficient width of the alveolar ridge, especially in the maxillary left lateral incisor (22) area to enable implant placement.

CASE DESCRIPTION

History

The patient had a clear medical history. There was no family history of hypodontia. She was a regular attendee at her general dentist. At the time of attendance at the multidisciplinary hypodontia clinic, she had completed fixed orthodontic appliance therapy and had been in orthodontic retention for 1 year. She was a non-anxious patient and she had undergone no other dental treatment. She had no parafunctional or nail-biting habits.

Oral hygiene was very good. She brushed twice daily with an adult-dose fluoride toothpaste.

Examination

The patient had denture stomatitis associated with the orthodontic retainer. The remaining soft tissues were healthy. She was caries-free.

The patient had gingival hyperplasia on the palatal aspect of the maxillary canines and first premolars. There was also an excess of gingival tissue on the ridges on the lateral incisor areas; this was severe enough to require crown lengthening. She was slightly short of space, mesiodistally for a lateral incisor implant. On palpation of the labial aspect of the alveolar ridge, there was a bony defect high up in the maxillary right lateral incisor (12) region.

The patient had a skeletal Class I relationship with a Class I (neutro) incisor relationship.

Additional Investigations

A panoramic radiograph confirmed the absence of the maxillary right and left lateral incisors (12, 22) and the mandibular right and left third molars (38, 48) (Fig. 6-1). Long cone periapicals of the upper incisor area showed good root parallelism and insufficient bone in the maxillary right lateral incisor (12) region (Fig. 6-2).

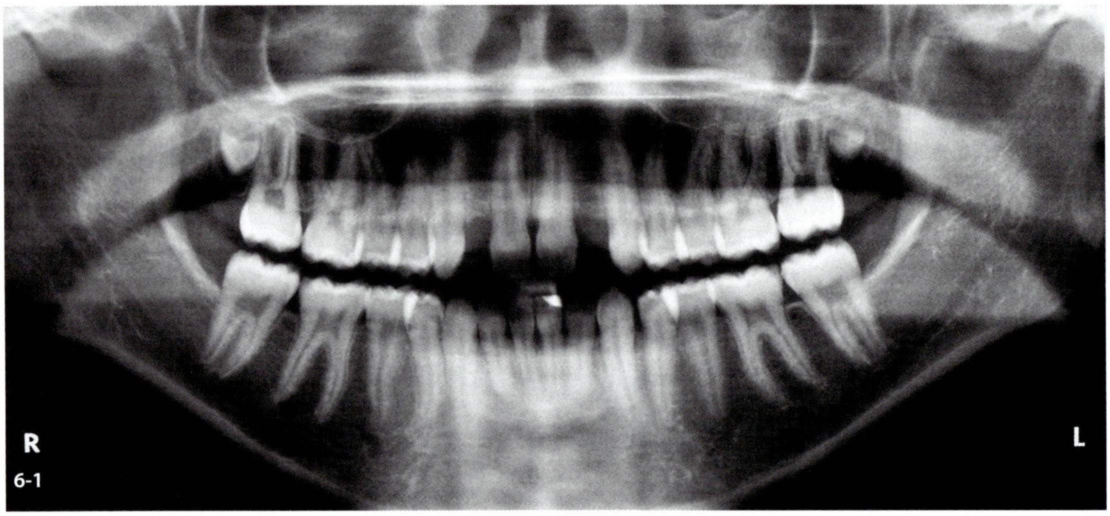

6-1

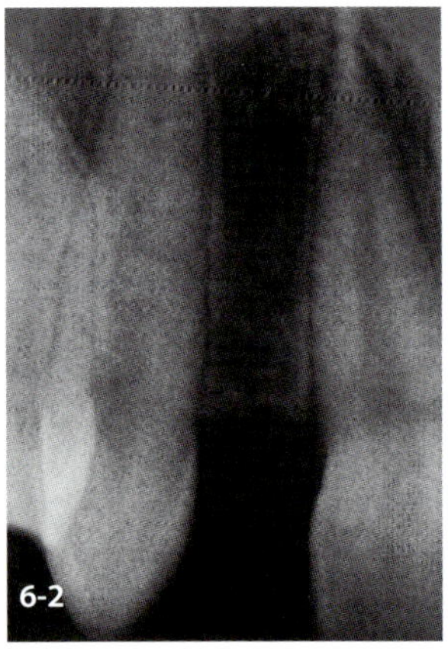
6-2

Fig. 6-1 Panoramic radiograph of a 14-year-old patient with congenitally missing maxillary lateral incisors, following orthodontic space opening.

Fig. 6-2 Periapical radiograph showing the alveolar bone in the maxillary lateral incisor region and root paralleling of the adjacent teeth.

DIAGNOSIS

Congenitally missing teeth – in this case, the maxillary lateral incisors and lower third molars.

TREATMENT OPTIONS

The aim of treatment was to restore the space in the maxillary right and left lateral incisor regions.

Definitive

- Resin-retained bridges were selected as the treatment of choice in this situation.

Alternatives

The alternative treatments were: partial denture, implants, and tooth transplantation.

- Partial dentures were ruled out since the patient was not keen to wear a removable prosthesis for an indefinite period.
- Implants placement is dependent on there being sufficient alveolar bone. Indeed, alveolar ridge augmentation is commonly required, for instance in cases of hypodontia in the lower incisor area. The bone graft is usually taken from the iliac crest. In the maxilla, it is not always feasible to heighten the alveolar ridge. Implantation is most commonly performed after growth has ceased. This patient was still a little too young to consider this, and there was inadequate space and bone for implants. Approximately, 1.5 mm of extra space is required mesiodistally for implant placement; this varies between implant systems.
- Tooth transplantation is an option where there is spacing in one region of the mouth and crowding in another. Mandibular second premolars are the most common choice for transplantation. Ideally, root formation should be between two-thirds to three-quarters. In the present case the patient had no crowding.

Rationale

The restorative solution was simpler and less invasive but still did not prevent implantation being considered in the future. Resin-retained bridges were selected because it was a conservative and simple choice for this patient and would probably produce the best esthetics. Resin-retained bridges have a good survival record[5] and have been shown to be effective in this clinical situation. However, their success is dependent on good planning, preparation, and lack of occlusal interference. There was no occlusal interference in this case and the patient had good canine guidance.

TREATMENT AND FOLLOW-UP

Treatment

The resin-retained bridges were bonded to the canines. The canines are most commonly selected because they offer the greatest surface area and there is less chance of 'shine-through' from the metal wings.

Since there was gingival overgrowth and inflammation in the canine and premolar areas, the patient was first placed on a hygiene program with a dental therapist, totalling four visits, and shown how to clean this area more efficiently. She was taught the Bass Technique, and interdental "TP" brushes (orange/blue; TePe) (Fig. 6-3) were used in the maxillary right and left canine and first premolar (13, 14, 23, 24) regions. Chlorhexidine gel was also used on the single tufted brush on the palatal surfaces of the maxillary right and left central incisors (11, 21). At the end of this treatment, gingival inflammation had reduced, although there was still some gingival overgrowth present on the maxillary right and left central incisors and canines (11, 13, 21, 23).

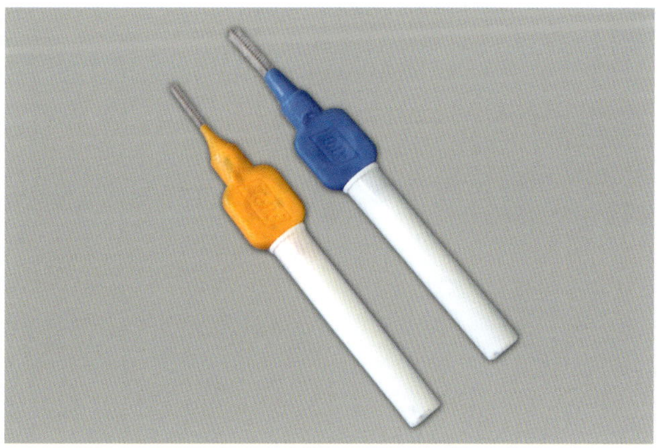

Fig. 6-3 Interdental brushes (TePe).

Alginate impressions were taken for a special tray. Gingival cautery was undertaken to remove the excess tissue from the palatal gingivae of the maxillary right and left canines (13, 23) and from the labial aspect of the ridge of the maxillary lateral incisors (12, 22). A finish line was prepared on the palatal aspects of the maxillary canines (13, 23) corresponding to the newly formed gingival margin. A silicone impression was made (Extrude) using the special tray. A lower alginate impression and a wax occlusal registration were taken. Shade (Vita) A2 with A1 with translucency at the incisal tip was selected for the pontic.

Local anesthetic was administered (20% benzocaine topical and 2.2. mL of 2% lidocaine with 1:80 000 adrenaline) to the palatal gingivae. The resin-retained bridges were first tried in using calcium hydroxide paste (Dycal) and the color, fit, and occlusion were checked. The patient was happy with the appearance. The bridges were then removed and the fitting areas sandblasted. The teeth were isolated using cotton wool rolls.

Gingival retraction cord was inserted, mainly palatally. The Panavia-XS system was used to cement the bridges. This involved etching the enamel surface with Panavia etch agent V for 15 seconds followed by application of the primer. The tooth surfaces were then air dried. Panavia 21 (tooth colored) was then applied to the metal wings and the bridges were seated. Excess cement was removed and the antioxidant applied. The retraction cord was removed together with the seating tag (Figs 6-4a to 6-4c, Fig. 6-5).

The patient was provided with Essix retainers (Fig. 6-6) to be worn at night. She was shown how to use Superfloss™ beneath the pontic and oral hygiene was reinforced.

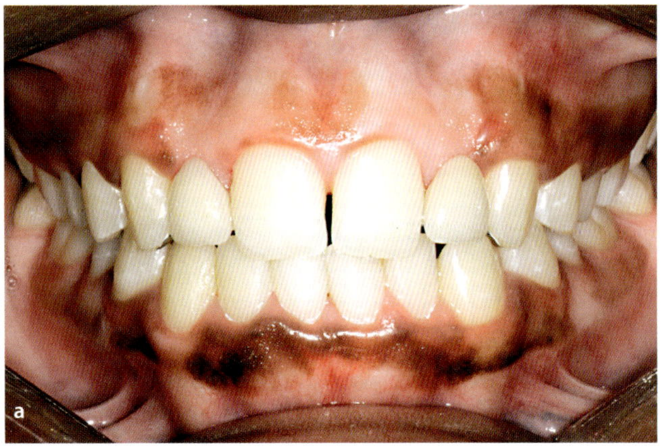

a

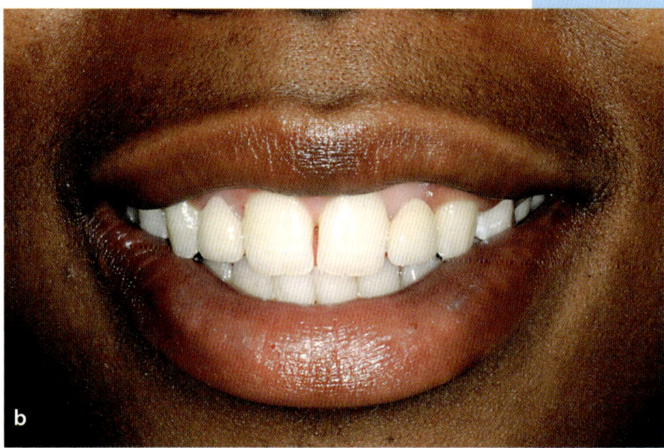

b

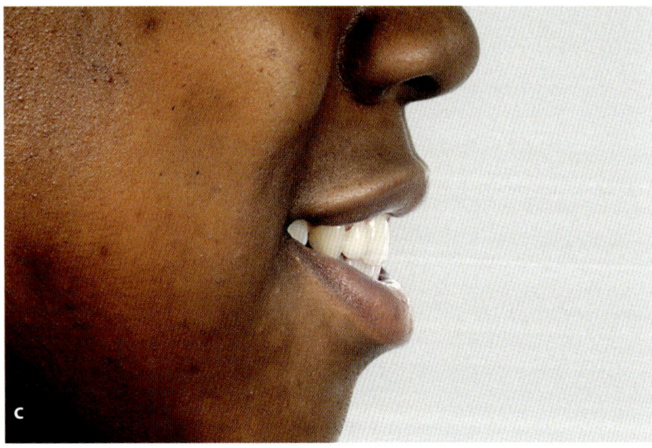

c

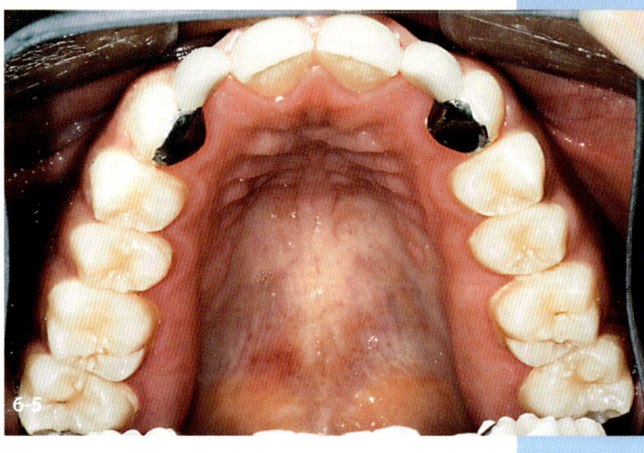

6-5

Fig. 6-4a–c Final result with two Maryland bridges.

Fig. 6-5 Occlusal view of the two bridges.

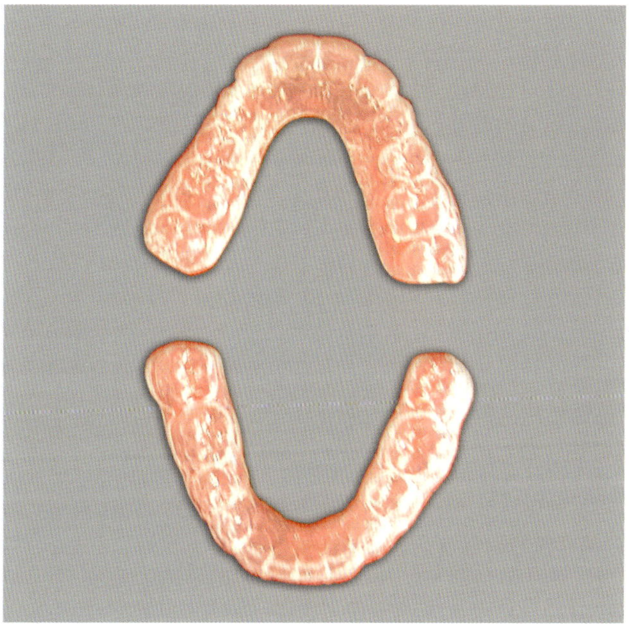

Fig. 6-6 Essix retainers.

> ***Key Message***
> *Canines are most commonly selected for resin-retained bridge abutments because they offer the greatest surface area and there is less chance of 'shine-through' from the metal wing.*

Posttreatment Evaluation/Follow-up

At the 3-month review, it was found that the Essix retainer had not been worn and the teeth had moved. However, the bridges were still intact and in a good position. A new retainer was provided and the importance of wear reinforced.

One year later, the patient was satisfied with the appearance of her teeth. On examination, oral hygiene was good but there was food packing under the bridges so the use of Superfloss was reinforced. She confirmed that the retainer was still being worn; this was demonstrated by the fact that it fitted well.

DISCUSSION

Tooth development, like the development of all epithelial tissues, is regulated by complex interactions between the epithelium and mesenchyme. A number of different mesenchymal molecules and their receptors act as mediators of the interactions during tooth development. These include the bone morphogenetic proteins and fibroblast growth factor (FGF). In dental mesenchyme, tooth development and shape is regulated by FGF8 and FGF9 via downstream factors Msh homeobox 1 (MSX1) and paired box gene 9 (PAX9).

Dental management is dependent on the child's compliance and attitude, pattern of missing teeth, the location of the spacing, and the malocclusion. All children will require dietary advice and oral hygiene instruction, especially when orthodontic appliances or dentures are in use. At least 1000 ppm fluoride toothpaste is recommended. Permanent molars should be fissure sealed. Regular review is important, and since they can be regarded as high caries risk, fluoride varnish may be applied every 3–4 months.[6]

It is important to consider the following when deciding which restorative option would be most appropriate for the patient: their preference, medical history, quality of abutment teeth, retention requirements, upper lip line and emergence profile. An implant could be considered; however, this will be governed by the quality and quantity of bone (an alveolar bone graft may be necessary), adjacent root position and angulation, interocclusal space, and the soft tissues.

Spacing, especially in the maxillary incisor area, is a common complaint of children with hypodontia. The clinical question is simple: should the space be maintained or closed? Space maintenance can be achieved by orthodontic appliances, partial dentures or by temporary adhesive bridges but can be difficult in the growing child, and so regular monitoring is essential. Preservation of the center-line and prevention of overeruption is also of paramount importance. It is particularly important to avoid overeruption of a mandibular canine into a maxillary incisor space.

Space closure can be achieved through both timely extraction of primary teeth and by orthodontic appliance therapy. Indeed, whatever the decision, orthodontic treatment may be required to position the remaining teeth, especially those that might later have a useful role as denture or bridge abutments. However, it is important that this orthodontic treatment is also planned as part of a multidisciplinary approach so that the space is adequate, unlike the case presented here.

Maxillary Lateral Incisor Spacing

Special mention should be made of the situation, such as this present case, where there is a missing maxillary lateral incisor. If space closure is considered, the canine could be reshaped to look like the missing incisor using direct or indirect composite veneers. This often appears to be the simpler solution in a growing child. However, this is dependent on the color and the shape and size of the canine. Some patients with hypodontia have large round canines that are difficult to camouflage. Moreover, the canine's emergence angle is different and the gingival margin is more apical than the maxillary incisors. Therefore, those who have high smile lines will not necessarily have a satisfactory esthetic result.

It is more common to consider space maintenance, or reopening, especially when complex restoration treatment such as adhesive bridges and implants are indicated. In cases such as these, it is most often best to keep the canines in their correct position to ensure canine guidance. However, the maxillary canines frequently erupt ectopically when lateral incisors are missing. It is commonly thought that the maxillary lateral incisor acts as a guide for canine eruption. In these cases, surgical exposure and orthodontic alignment is also required in advance of the definitive restorative treatment.

Key Message

Children and adolescents with hypodontia need emotional support, esthetic management, and multidisciplinary treatment planning for successful pediatric dental care.

ACKNOWLEDGMENTS

The authors are grateful to Dr Martin Kelleher, Consultant in Restorative Dentistry, King's College London, for his thoughtful treatment planning and help in the management of this patient. The authors would also like to acknowledge the unending help and support of Mrs Joanne Hales in the preparation of this manuscript.

REFERENCES

1. Aasheim B, Ogaard B. Hypodontia in 9-year-old Norwegians related to need of orthodontic treatment. Scand J Dent Res 1993;101:257–260.
2. Brooks AH. Dental anomalies of number, form and size: their prevalence in British schoolchildren. J Int Assoc Dent Child 1974;5:37–53.
3. Nunn JH, Carter ME, Gillgrass TJ, Hobson RS, Jepson NJ, Meechan JG, et al. The interdisciplinary management of hypodontia: background and the role of paediatric dentistry. Br Dent J 2003;194:245–251.
4. Hobkirk JA, Goodman JR, Jones SP. Presenting complaints and findings in a group of patients attending a hypodontia clinic. Br Dent J 1994;177:337–339.
5. Creugers NHJ, Kayser AF, Vant Hof MA. A seven and a half year survival study of resin bonded bridges. J Dent Res 1992;71:1822–1825.
6. Scottish Intercollegiate Guidelines Network. Targeted prevention of dental caries in the permanent teeth of 6–16 year olds presenting for dental care 2000. SIGN 47. Edinburgh: Royal College of Physicians of Edinburgh.

7

Erosive Dental Wear

Marie-Charlotte Huysmans
Gert Stel

Key words: tooth wear, dental erosion, erosive wear

Age category: 7–12 years

Definition

Dental erosion is defined as the loss of dental hard tissue due to chemical dissolution of the tooth surface by acids without bacterial involvement. The acids may be of intrinsic origin, ie, gastric acid entering the mouth for instance during vomiting, or of extrinsic origin, eg, dietary acids in soft drinks or citrus fruit. Recently it has been recognized that dental erosion modifies the mechanical types of wear, such as attrition and abrasion, and the term "erosive dental wear" has been proposed for the multifactorial process of dental wear in the presence of acid challenges. Due to differences in diagnostic criteria, the reported prevalence of erosive dental wear among children varies widely. However, epidemiologic evidence is now available showing that it may be a growing problem.[1]

THE PROBLEM

Ray (age 10) was referred by his dentist for extreme wear of his primary molars and canines. In all the affected teeth, the occlusal/incisal enamel was completely lost and the dentin exposed. The wear extended beyond the antagonistic contact areas, and there was a distinct "washed-out" appearance of the dentinal areas (Figs 7-1a, 7-1b). The patient had not experienced any caries and had no restorations.

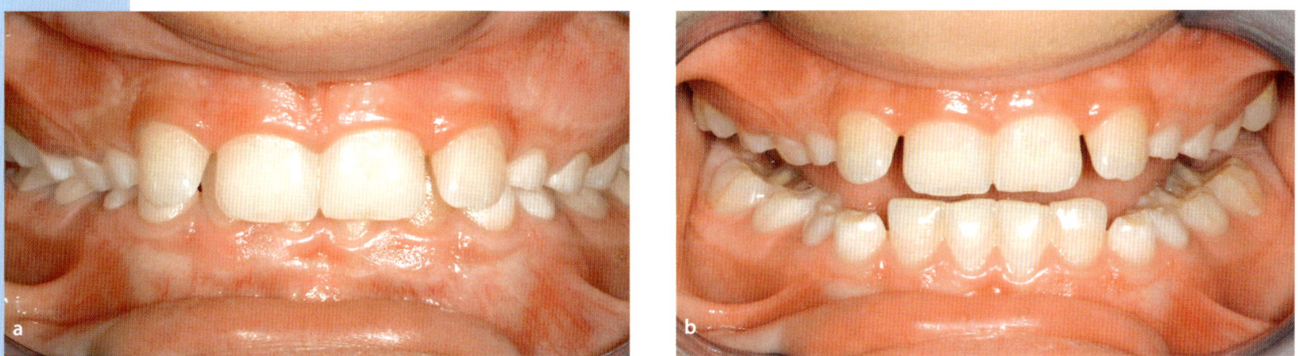

Fig. 7-1 A 10-year-old boy, referred to the university dental clinic for treatment of erosive dental wear. Anterior facial view in 7-1a habitual occlusion and 7-1b with the mouth slightly open.

CASE DESCRIPTION

History

Ray was the second child in a complete family. He was attending primary school and planning a presentation on dental erosion. His older sister had gastroesophageal reflux disease (GORD). When he played football with his team, they would drink lemonade in the breaks. Ray liked to eat sweet things and apples, and drank about two glasses of soft drinks (fruit based or cola drinks) per day. He took a long time to drink a glass, but he did not keep the drink in his mouth for a long time. His teeth were never sore or sensitive after drinking soft drinks.

Medical History

ASA 1. Ray was in good health. As a baby he had had asthma-like complaints, which had improved over the years. Also in his first years, GORD had been suspected but not confirmed. He had experienced a period of eczema, which had resolved completely. He had hoarseness now and then but no problems with swallowing food.

> ***Key Message***
> *In cases of erosive dental wear, always consider the possibility of reflux disease.*

Dental History

Ray had been visiting the dentist regularly, twice a year, since the age of 2 years. Only preventive intervention had been necessary. No caries activity was observed. Recently, the excessive wear of his primary dentition had been noticed, the subject of possible dental erosion was discussed, and a year later he was referred to the university dental clinic for diagnosis and treatment.

Oral Hygiene

Oral hygiene was good. Ray brushed his teeth twice a day with a fluoride-containing toothpaste aimed at restoring the oral pH balance.

Examination

Ray's muscles of mastication did not seem to be abnormally tense. He had a complete mixed dentition, up to the first permanent molars. The permanent incisors were in deep overbite, or "cover-bite", position.

There was substantial loss of tissue in the primary teeth, especially in the maxillary teeth. The canines were worn by about 50%, and the maxillary first primary molars showed complete enamel loss and scooped-out loss of dentin (Figs 7-2a, 7-2b). In the permanent teeth, signs of early enamel loss were already present. The permanent molars showed some loss of occlusal morphology and visual outlining of the dentin core. In the maxillary central incisors some palatal and incisal enamel smoothing was seen, as well as in the lower central incisors on the labial aspect. Wear facets were visible on the permanent molars and also on the incisors, although less well demarcated on the latter (Figs 7-3a to 7-3c). The teeth were not sensitive, and there were no signs of caries.

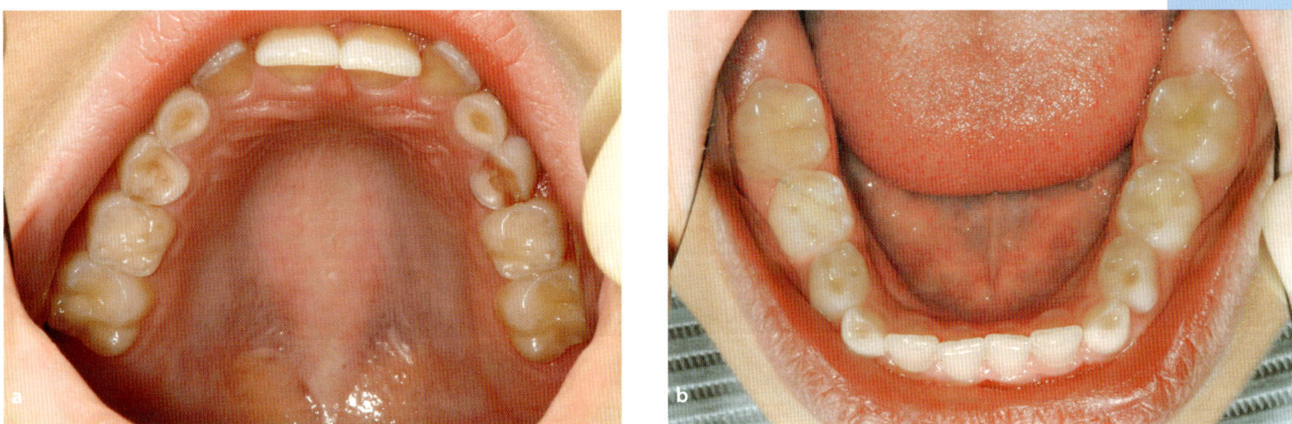

Fig. 7-2a,b Occlusal views of the maxillary and mandibular teeth. Note the extreme wear on the maxillary canines and first primary molars. Note the scooped-out appearance of the cusps of the lower primary molars.

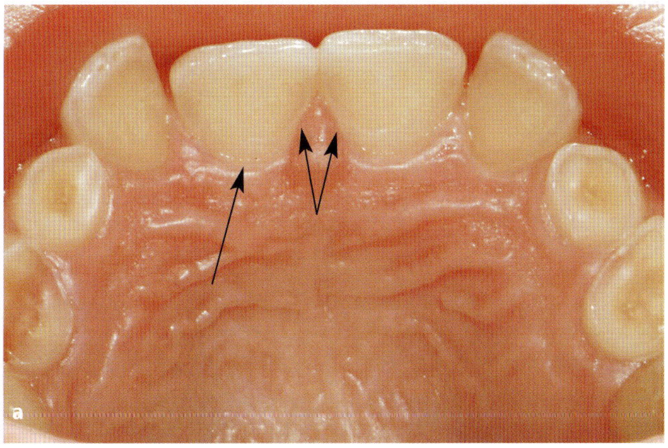

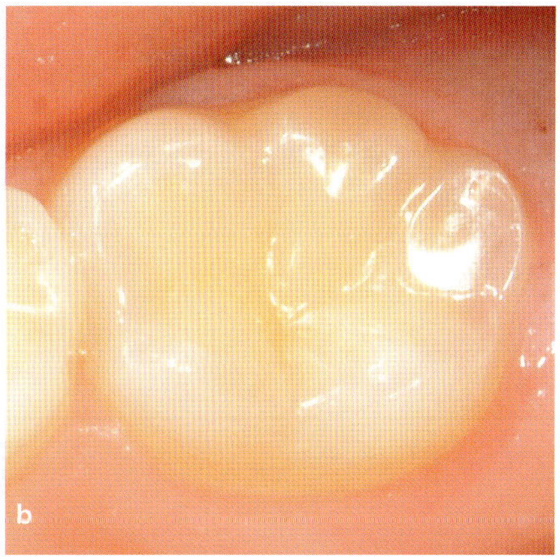

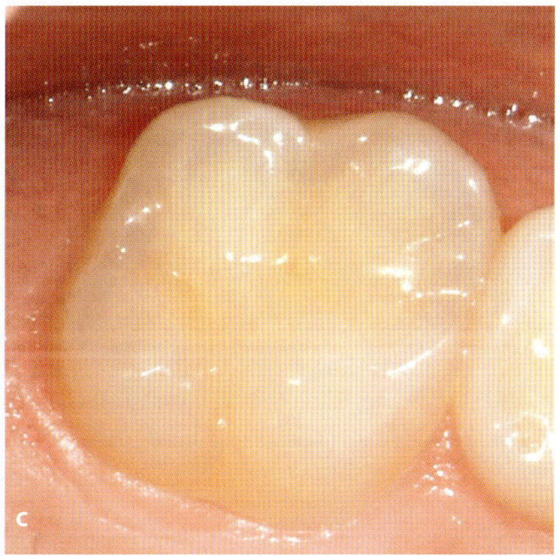

Fig. 7-3 Detailed views of some of the teeth. 7-3a The palatal surfaces of the maxillary incisors have a ridge at the gingival margin, where plaque or sulcular fluid protects the enamel (single arrow) and the outline of the dentin core is visible (double arrow). 7-3b The mandibular first molar has large wear facets. 7-3c The outline of the dentin core is visible on the maxillary first molar. Both molars show some loss of occlusal morphology.

Additional Investigations

Ray and his parents were asked to keep a dietary diary for 5 days. The diary showed that the patient had an acceptable eating and drinking frequency: about seven times a day, a little more often in the weekends. His favorite snacks were sweet things and his soft drink consumption was a bit higher than he thought: he drank orange-based drinks and sports drinks two to four times a day, not including milk-based drinks. Previous dietary advice by their own dentist had resulted in this behavior, as Ray's parents indicated that his frequency of intake of soft drinks had been even higher before.

Key Message

When assessing etiological factors of tooth wear, always make use of a dietary diary and ask about habits such as holding drinks in the mouth for a long time, or rinsing with them.

Besides the more usual causal factors, such as soft drinks, also consider less common ones. Acidic candies, eg, candy spray or gels, can induce a rapid decrease of salivary pH, sometimes even below pH 5, and are therefore potentially erosive.[2]

Salivary tests showed that the patient had rather low rate of salivary flow: 0.18 mL/min unstimulated flow, and 0.6 mL/min chewing stimulated flow. His salivary buffering capacity was medium. His parents decided against investigations for GORD, on the grounds of insufficient evidence for its involvement to justify the invasive procedure.

Diagnosis of dental erosive wear in this case was mainly based on the extent and the characteristics of the observed wear: smooth borders, loss of morphology, scooped-out dentin ("cupping", Fig. 7-4). However, in this case there was also a clear indication for tooth–tooth contacts to be of importance: the wear facets on the permanent molars and the labial wear of the mandibular incisors because of the cover-bite contacts. The erosive challenges soften the enamel surface, thus potentiating the wear effect of attritional forces.

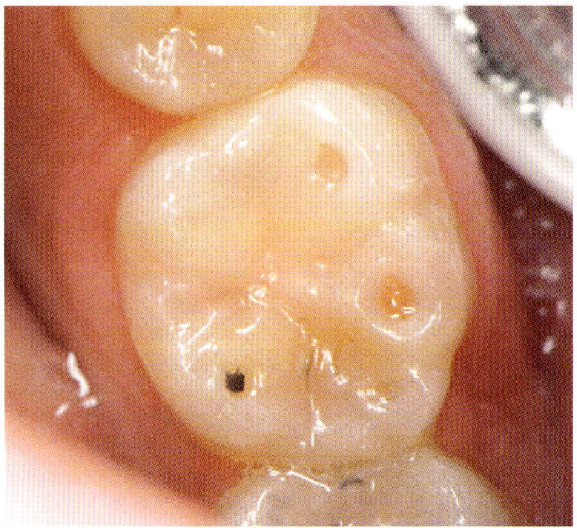

Fig. 7-4 A mandibular permanent molar in an unrelated case showing "cupping" lesions of the buccal cusps.

The etiology in this case was thus quite complicated. Three possible contributing factors may be considered:

- frequent exposure to dietary acids in soft drinks
- possible gastric reflux
- low salivary flow.

TREATMENT AIM

- To stop the progression of dental erosive wear by reducing the erosive challenges and enhancing the oral defence mechanism.
- If causation is still doubtful, extra attention to be given to dental hard tissue protection.

TREATMENT OPTIONS

- Dietary advice
- General health advice
- Oral hygiene advice

Rationale

Primary prevention of erosive wear involves reduction of the erosive challenges; in our patient's case this was especially the reduction in the frequency of soft drink intake. Secondly, the dental hard tissues must be protected. Unlike in the prevention of caries – where lower doses of fluoride might be effective – for erosive wear both the concentration and acidity of the fluoride-containing preventive product are different. Intensive fluoridation with high fluoride concentration/low pH formulations seems to be promising. A 1.25% fluoride gel was shown to be effective in a clinical model.[3] Owing to the acidic pH, superficial enamel dissolves and large amounts of calcium fluoride precipitate, delaying enamel dissolution during the next erosive challenge.

Preventive treatment

- Dietary advice: reduction of soft drink intake to ≤2 times/day.
- General health advice: monitor signs of reflux disease (GORD).
- Oral hygiene/fluoride advice: brush with fluoride gel (Elmex®, GABA International) one to two times per week.

TREATMENT AND FOLLOW-UP

Treatment

Very little is known about the natural history of erosive dental wear and the clinical effectiveness of preventive measures. Very few longitudinal studies are available, and none at all have evaluated clinical preventive treatment. Therefore, our patient's prognosis is not known. Treatment is ongoing with regular monitoring of the preventive regimen. Periodic checkups will be necessary to evaluate the efficacy of the preventive measures.

Posttreatment Evaluation/Follow-up

Monitoring the subtle changes to the dentition in erosive wear can be difficult. One way of registering change is to make use of both clinical intraoral photographs and radiographs.[1] Study models/casts made at regular intervals can also be helpful in the monitoring process (Figs 7-5a, 7-5b).

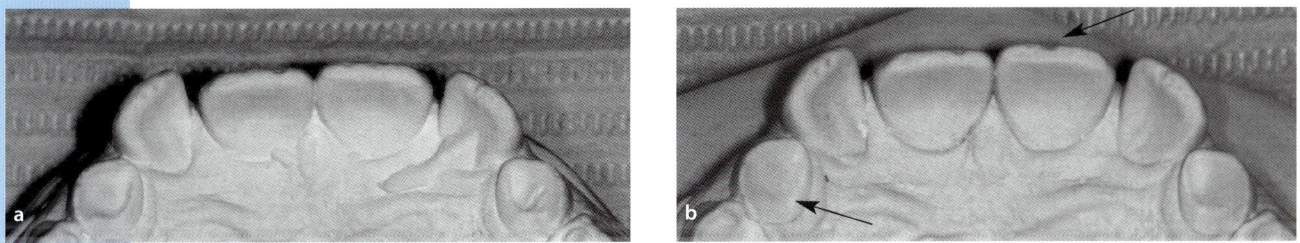

Fig. 7-5 Detailed view of stone models of the maxillary dentition. 7-5a One year before the consultation. 7-5b Situation at consultation. Note the subtle indications of continued wear.

DISCUSSION

The term GORD is used to describe symptoms of mucosal damage resulting from gastric acid and pepsin; however, reflux is often asymptomatic ("silent refluxers"). Besides the more obvious signs of GORD, such as an acidic taste in the mouth or vomiting, there are more subtle signs, including: hoarseness, difficulty swallowing, coughing, experiencing a "lump" in the throat.

GORD is a common condition affecting approximately 35–40% of the Western population.[5] The prevalence among children is estimated to be between 1.8% and 22%.[6] Dental erosion is more prevalent among GORD patients, with a median prevalence of 17% (range 14–87%).[7] Asthma has also been identified as a risk factor for dental erosion. Several hypotheses for this relationship have been proposed, such as the low pH of powder inhalers. However, there is also evidence that GORD, which is often associated with asthma, is the intermediate factor in erosion in asthmatic people.[8]

It is not always easy to differentiate between dental erosive wear and physiological wear of dental hard tissues. Different etiological factors may be involved. A concise definition of different tooth surface lesions can be helpful in determining etiological factors and therapeutic measures.[9] At a mean age of 5 in about a third of children, primary teeth display incisal and/or occlusal wear[10] (Fig. 7-6). Since the severity and the number of affected teeth can vary considerably, early diagnosis is necessary, especially in patients in whom erosion of the primary teeth is considered to be a predictor for erosion and generalized wear of the permanent dentition.[11]

Normal wear and tear of primary teeth rarely leads to discomfort or dysfunctional problems; occasionally, excessive wear may cause occlusal effects, eg, crossbites and/or negative overbites. These occur in about 5% of children in the age group of 6–8 years.[12] Early orthodontic intervention may be necessary. Restorative treatment is indicated only in exceptional cases. Worn deciduous molars that are sensitive often cannot easily be restored with intraoral restorations. The placement of stainless steel crowns, however, can be a satisfactory way of providing relief of symptoms and cessation of continued wear. Also it is more likely that normal exfoliation will occur.[13] When permanent teeth are involved, the decision to commence preventive and/or restorative interventional treat-

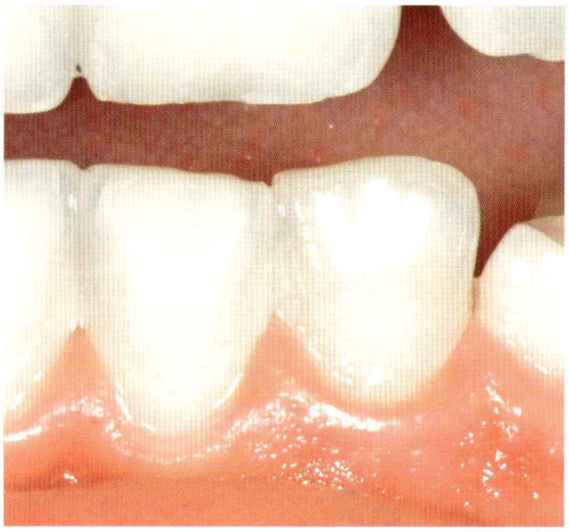

Fig. 7-6 Example of physiologic wear of the primary dentition.

ment should be based on clinical considerations. When the patient has severe discomfort, such as pain, or complains about poor esthetics and/or functional disturbances, restorative intervention is advised. In our patient none of these circumstances were present, and restorative treatment was not yet indicated. The treatment of choice will depend on both the patient and the operator and the feasibility of altering etiological factors. Resin composites are generally considered first choice, because of their minimally invasive characteristics.

Key Messages

Early diagnosis allows for early preventive intervention. Early signs include:

- *polished appearance of the tooth surfaces, with loss of incremental lines*
- *loss of sharpness/smoothing of tooth contours*
- *visibility of the yellow dentin core*
- *cupping of cusps.*

REFERENCES

1. Truin GJ, van Rijkom HM, Mulder J, van't Hof MA. Caries trends 1996-2002 among 6- and 12-year-old children and erosive wear prevalence among 12-year-old children in The Hague. Caries Res 2005;39:2–8.
2. Gambon DL, Keijbus PAM van den, Nieuw Amerongen A van. Candy sprays and gels: effect on salivary flow and pH. Ned Tijdschr Tandheelk 2006;113:27–32.
3. Ganss C, Klimek J, Brune V, Schürmann A. Effects of two fluoridation measures on erosion progression in human enamel and dentine in situ. Caries Res 2004;38:561–566.
4. Al-Malik MI, Holt RD, Bedi R, Speight PM. Investigation of an index to measure tooth wear in primary teeth. J Dent 2001;29:103–107.
5. Farrokhi F, Vaezi MF. Extra-esophageal manifestations of gastroesophageal reflux. Oral Dis 2007;13:349–359.
6. Hassall E. Decisions in diagnosing and managing chronic gastroesophageal reflux disease in children. J Pediatr 2005;146:S3–12.
7. Pace F, Pallotta S, Tonini M, Vakil N, Bianchi Porro G. Systematic review: gastro-oesophageal reflux disease and dental lesions. Aliment Pharmacol Ther 2008;27:1179–1186.
8. Sivasithamparam K, Young WG, Jirattanasopa V, Priest J, Khan F, Harbrow D, et al. Dental erosion in asthma: a case-control study from south east Queensland. Austr Dent J 2002;47:298–303.
9. Grippo JO, Simring M, Schreiner S. Attrition, abrasion, corrosion and abfraction revisited: A new perspective on tooth surface lesions. J Am Dent Assoc 2004;135:1109–1118.
10. Hugoson A, Ekfeldt A, Koch G, Hallonsten AL. Incisal and occlusal tooth wear in children and adolescents in a Swedish population. Acta Odontol Scand 1996;54:263–270.
11. Ganss C, Klimek J, Giese K. Dental erosion in children and adolescents – a cross-sectional and longitudinal investigation using study models. Community Dent Oral Epidemiol 2001;29:264–271.
12. Tausche E, Luck O, Harzer W. Prevalence of malocclusions in the early mixed dentition and orthodontic treatment need. Eur J Orthod 2004;26:237–244.
13. Harley K. Tooth wear in the child and the youth. Br Dent J 1999;186:492–496.

8

The Hall Technique: A Novel Method of Using Preformed Metal Crowns

Nicola Innes
Dafydd Evans

Key words: Hall technique, dental anxiety, hypoplastic, hypomineralized primary molars, carious primary molars, preformed metal crowns

Age category: 4–7 years

Definition
The Hall technique is a method of managing a primary molar that is carious or hypoplastic, using a preformed metal crown (PMC). With the Hall technique, the PMC is cemented onto the tooth, using a glass-ionomer cement, without the use of local anesthesia, caries removal or crown reduction. This differs from standard practice for fitting a PMC, where local anesthesia is achieved, carious tooth tissue is removed, and the tooth is prepared to receive the PMC (reduction of the mesial, distal and occlusal aspects of the crown with a high-speed rotary handpiece), which is then cemented into place.

Full clinical details of the Hall technique are available,[1] as are 2-year results from a randomized controlled clinical trial.[2] This report illustrates use of the Hall technique in managing developmental defects of enamel and carious primary molars in a young, anxious child.

THE PROBLEM

Alistair (aged 2¾ years) was referred by his general dental practitioner for management of his second primary molars (55, 65, 75, 85), which appeared to have a developmental defect of enamel, and were sensitive when being brushed. On examination, enamel hypoplasia with missing areas of enamel was diagnosed. Management of these teeth was complicated by the patient having difficulty in accepting any dental intervention, partly as a result of his young age. Maintenance of the teeth with oral hygiene alone was insufficient to prevent continued breakdown of the enamel surface, so PMCs were placed on the affected teeth, using the Hall technique (Hall crowns).

CASE DESCRIPTION

History

Medical History
ASA I. Alistair was fit and healthy. His mother reported that the pregnancy had reached term, and both the pregnancy and the birth had been uneventful. There was no remarkable medical history.

Dental History
When Alistair was nearly 3 years old (July 2003), his general dental practitioner referred him to the preventive and children's section at Dundee Dental Hospital and School because of the clinical appearance of all the second primary molars (55, 65, 75, 85). The teeth did not cause him any pain when he was eating, but were sensitive when brushed by his mother.

Examination

When Alistair attended the clinic for assessment, he expressed anxiety about even sitting in the dental chair. The clinical appearance of the second primary molars was of a developmental defect of enamel, with diffuse areas of opacities and hypoplasia. All four teeth showed evidence of posteruptive enamel breakdown. There were also some demarcated opacities visible on some other primary teeth, including the first primary molars and canines. It was not possible to take radiographs or photographs due to the poor level of cooperation. There were no signs or symptoms of irreversible pulpal disease affecting the second primary molars, and the hypoplastic areas had large areas of missing enamel but were relatively hard on probing. No dental caries was identified.

TREATMENT AIMS

The aims of treatment were to:

- relieve symptoms associated with brushing the second primary molars
- prevent further deterioration of the teeth
- encourage and develop a positive attitude in the patient toward dental treatment.

TREATMENT OPTIONS

Provisional

In view of the patient's poor level of cooperation, it was decided, in consultation with his mother, to initially manage the hypoplastic teeth with a preventive program: tooth brushing instruction, applications of fluoride varnish (Duraphat™, Colgate), and dietary advice. As cooperation improved, the second primary molars would be temporized with glass-ionomer cement until Alistair was able to accept a more permanent restorative option.

Definitive

Once adequate cooperation had been obtained, the second primary molars would be managed with PMCs.

Rationale

The second primary molars were causing Alistair only a minor problem, and he was very anxious about dental treatment. Therefore, the treatment priorities were to balance the effective management of the affected teeth (reducing the risk of continuing deterioration, resulting in further pain) against the risk of treatment-induced anxiety (through introducing invasive treatment before he was able to accept it). Intensive prevention, and applications of glass-ionomer cement, would allow him to become acclimatized to dental treatment, and also slow down the deterioration of the affected primary molars.

> ***Key Message***
> *The provision of dental care for young children may need to be staged in order to allow their ability to cooperate with treatment to develop. However, this must be balanced against managing any discomfort they are experiencing.*

TREATMENT AND FOLLOW-UP

Initially, treatment consisted of toothbrushing instruction with Alistair's mother, with the aim of keeping the hypoplastic areas of the molar teeth plaque-free. The use of warm water when brushing was recommended to reduce thermal sensitivity. In addition, fluoride varnish (Duraphat) was applied, following the Scottish national guideline (Scottish Intercollegiate Guidelines Network

[SIGN] 83).[3] Over the next 2 years, further deterioration of the second primary molars was noted, but the patient's cooperation did not improve sufficiently to allow the provision of definitive restorative care. Instead, treatment was limited to the temporization of all four second primary molars with glass-ionomer cement. However, there were considerable problems with moisture control, and the material was noted to be quickly lost.

Just before Alistair's fifth birthday, it was clear that the preventive program, and the use of glass-ionomer cement, was not preventing continued deterioration of the second primary molars, and that the provision of the definitive treatment of PMCs could not be delayed any further. However, the patient's cooperation, although improving, was still poor. Following discussion with the patient and his mother, it was felt that he would be able to tolerate the minimally invasive procedure of providing PMCs using the Hall technique. Hall crowns were cemented to both the maxillary primary second molars (55, 65) (the most severely affected teeth) using glass-ionomer cement (1 month apart). Alistair accepted this treatment well, and allowed photographs to be taken at a subsequent appointment (Figs 8-1a to 8-1e). Managing to cope fitting the Hall crowns increased his self-confidence, and he was then happy to accept Hall crowns on the mandibular primary second molars (75, 85) 1 month later. Figure 8-2 shows the steps in the placement of the Hall crown on the mandibular right primary second molar (85).

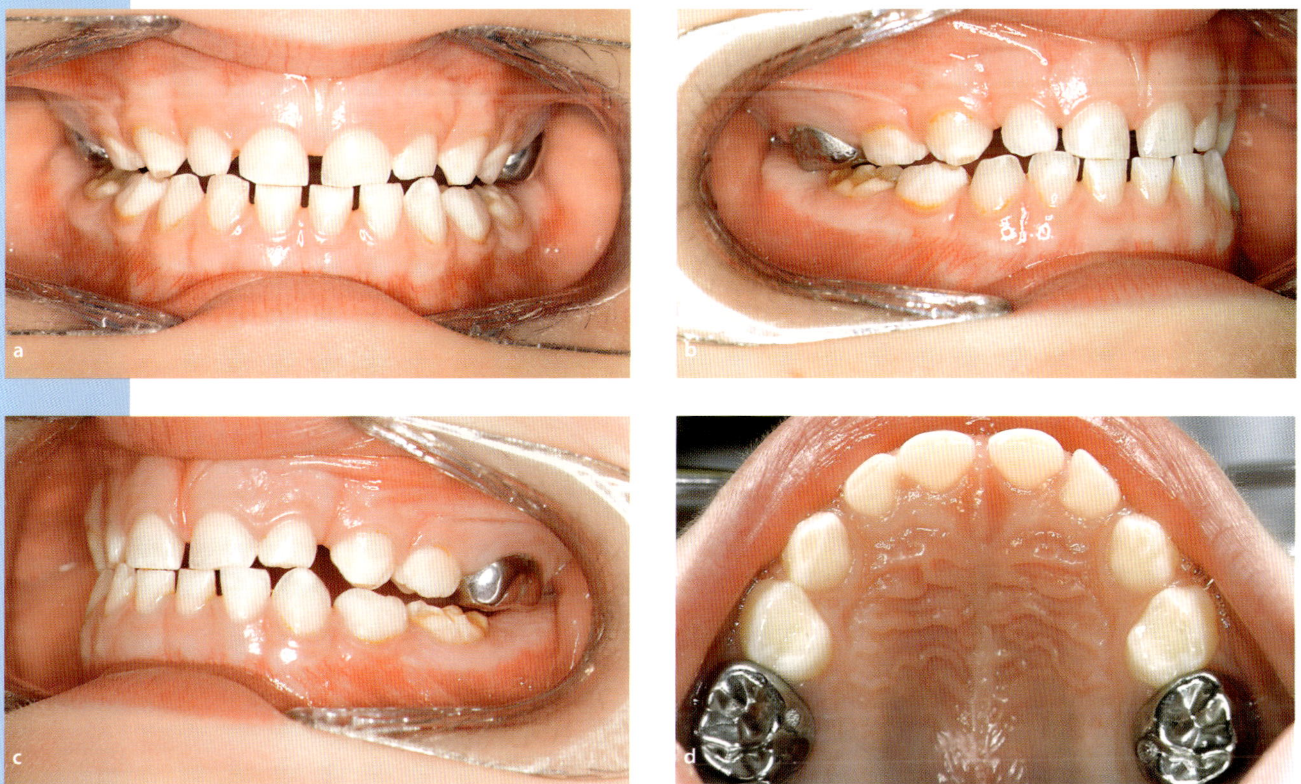

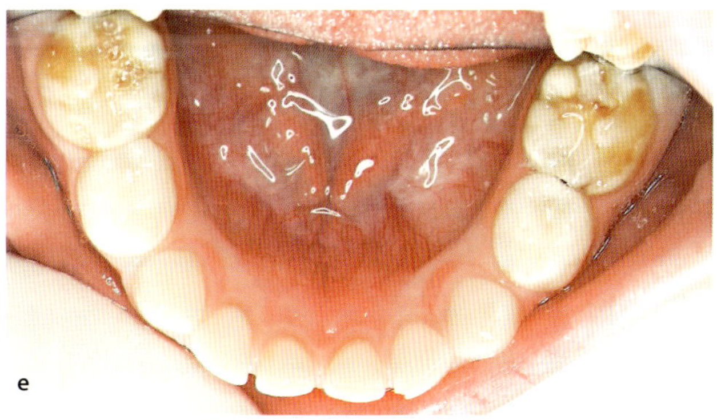

Fig. 8-1a–e Full mouth views taken aged 5 years and 2 months. Preformed metal crowns have already been fitted to the maxillary primary second molars (55, 65) (2 and 3 months previously). 8-1a–c Re-established occlusion (existing Class III molar relationship on the left side). 8-1d PMCs on maxillary primary second molars (55, 65). 8-1e The two hypoplastic second primary molars.

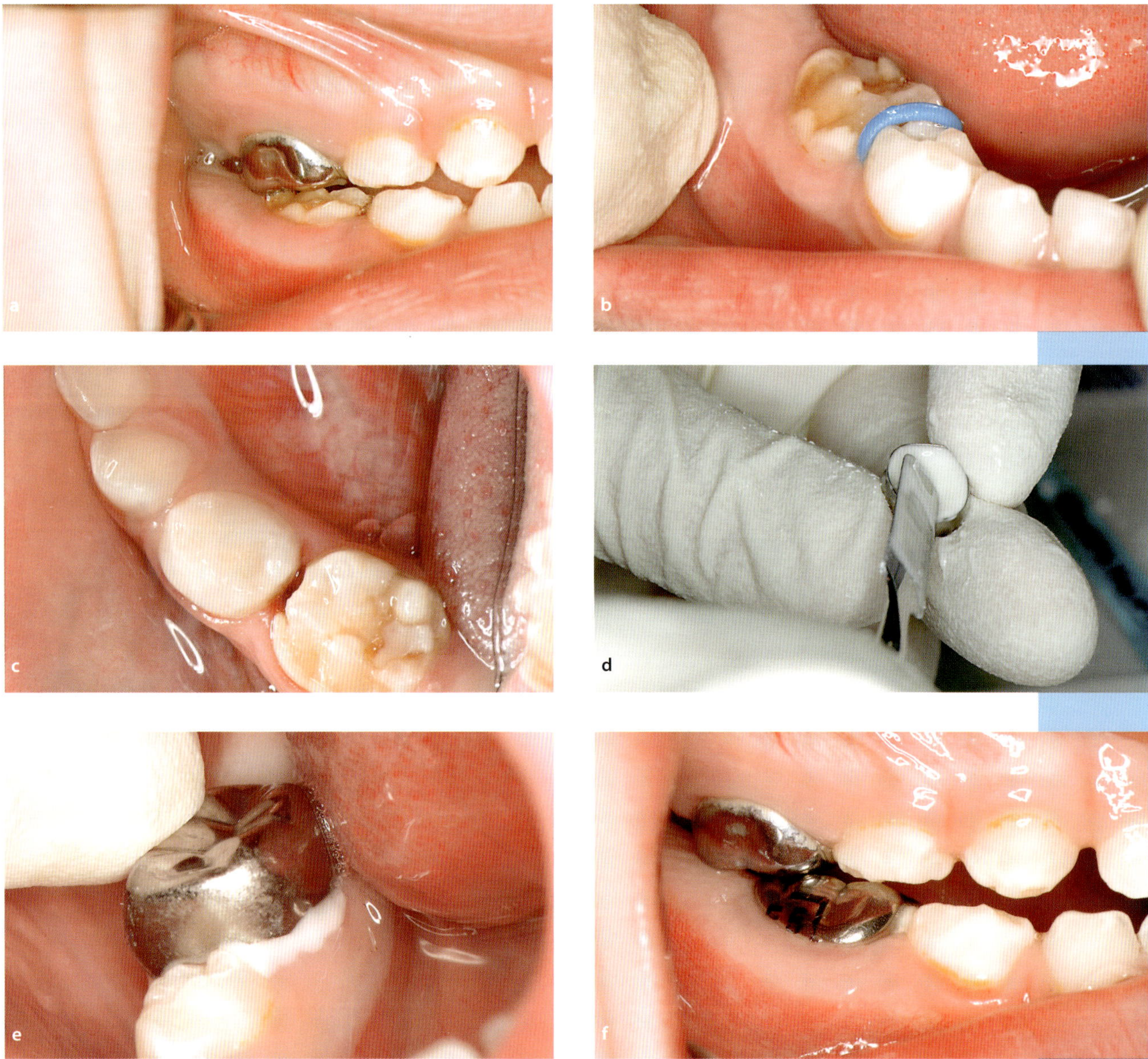

Fig. 8-2a–f Sequence for fitting Hall crown to the mandibular right primary second molar (85) with use of a separator to create space mesially. 8-2a Lateral view prior to fitting crown. 8-2b Separator placed. 8-2c Separator removed 5 days later, showing space. 8-2d Crown being filled with glass ionomer cement. 8-2e Crown being placed on tooth. 8-2f Crown fitted. Glass-ionomer will be removed from between the mandibular right primary molar (84, 85) using dental floss.

Four months after this, when Alistair was 5½ years of age, his cooperation had improved sufficiently to allow radiographs to be taken (Figs 8-3a, 8-3b). These showed caries affecting the maxillary left primary first molar (64) and the mandibular right primary first molar (84). Initially these lesions were managed with prevention alone, but as they were noted to be progressive, with new carious lesions developing on the maxillary right primary first molar (54) and the mandibular left primary first molar (74), Hall crowns were placed on all four first primary molars by the time the patient was 6 years of age (Fig. 8-4). Whereas composite restorations may have been considered more esthetic restorations for these teeth by the patient and his mother, they have not expressed any concern over the appearance of the crowns. Alistair was happy with the crowns and although his cooperation with treatment and ability to remain still in the dental chair were improving, it was unlikely that he would have tolerated four individual appointments with local anesthetic and use of rotary instruments. In addition, moisture control may well have been difficult to maintain, compromising the quality of the restorations.

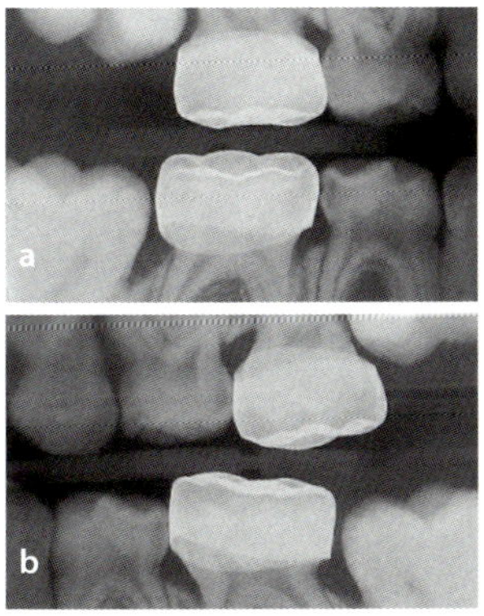

Fig. 8-3 Bitewing radiographs (age 5½ years). 8-3a Right bitewing radiograph; 8-3b left bitewing radiograph.

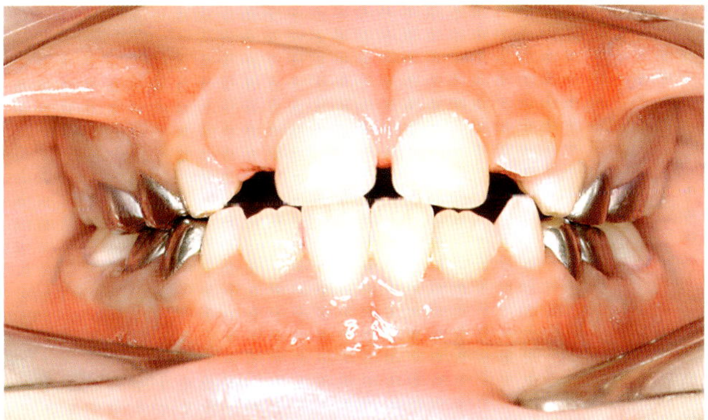

Fig. 8-4 Anterior view (age 6 years 2 months) showing equal occlusal contact on both sides and establishing permanent dentition.

As the patient was clearly at increased risk of dental caries, the partially erupted first permanent molars were fissure sealed with Fuji VII™ (GC) as a temporary measure, until they had erupted sufficiently to allow placement of resin sealants.

History, clinical examination, and bitewing radiographs (Figs 8-5a to 8-5d) at 7 years of age (2 years after the first, and 1 year after the last, Hall crowns were fitted) found no signs or symptoms of pulpal disease and no new carious lesions. Alistair's cooperation had also improved sufficiently to allow resin sealants to be placed on the first permanent molars.

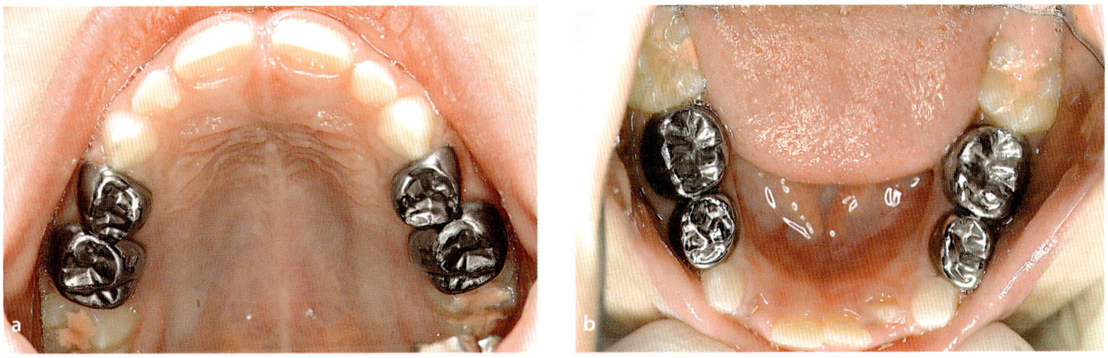

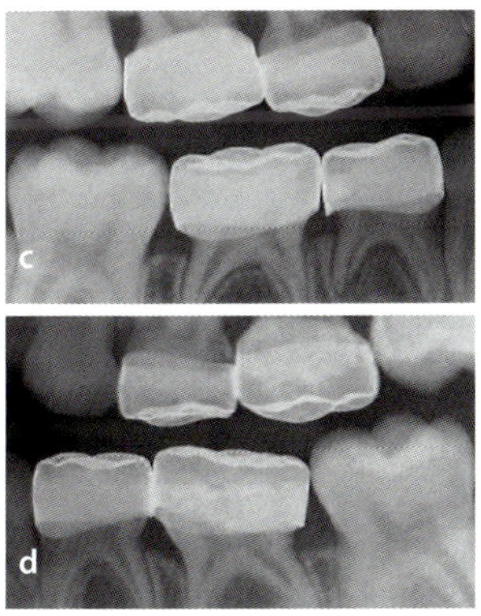

Fig. 8-5a–d Age 7 years. 8-5a,b Eight PMCs fitted using Hall technique and glass-ionomer temporary fissure sealants on the first permanent molars. 8-1c,d Right and left bitewing radiographs.

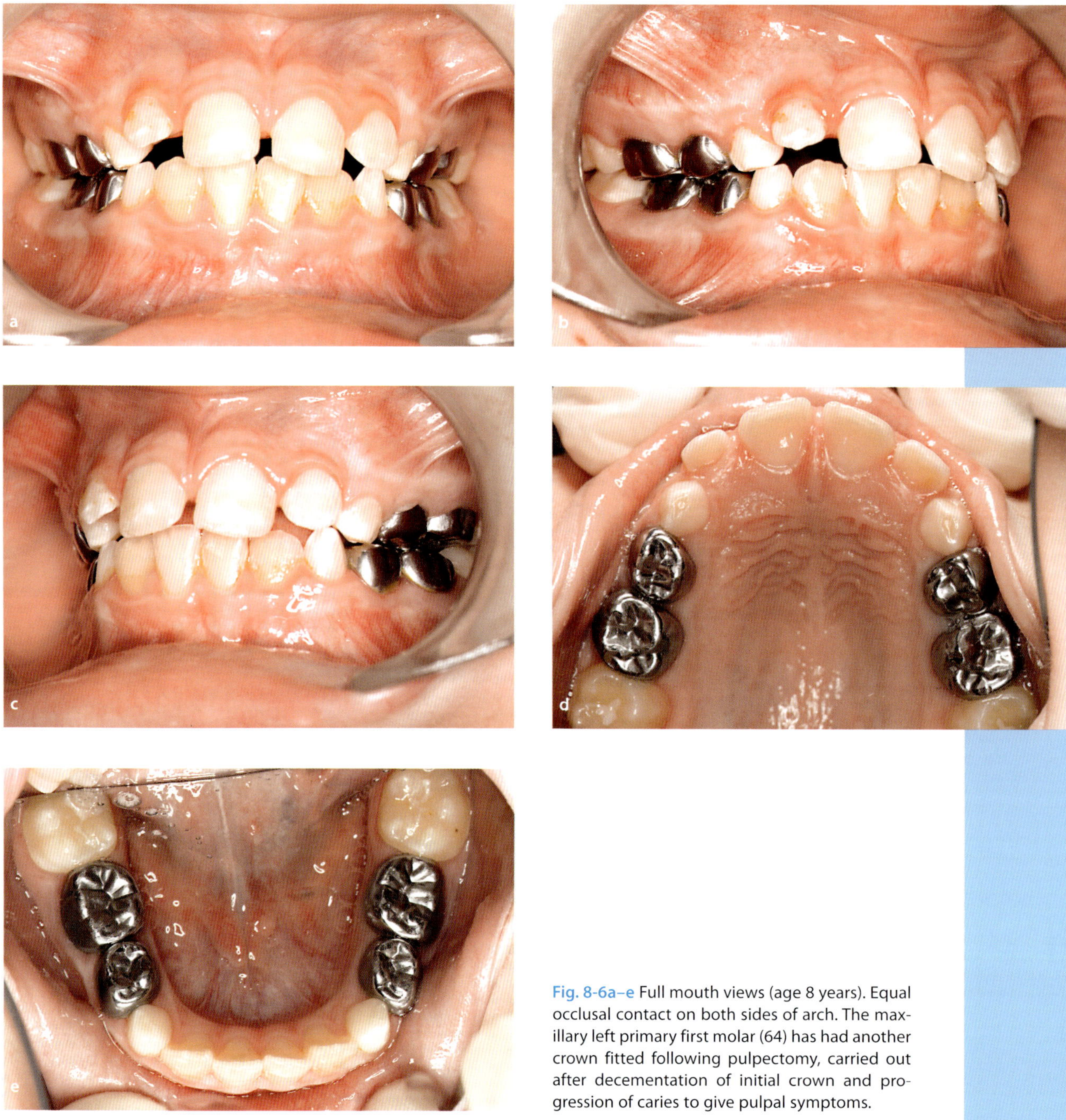

Fig. 8-6a–e Full mouth views (age 8 years). Equal occlusal contact on both sides of arch. The maxillary left primary first molar (64) has had another crown fitted following pulpectomy, carried out after decementation of initial crown and progression of caries to give pulpal symptoms.

At the patient's latest recall appointment, it was noted that the PMC on the maxillary left primary first molar (64) had decemented. The patient stated that it had been lost several months ago and the tooth had recently become painful. On clinical examination, a large mesio-occlusal carious lesion was noted on the tooth, which was tender to percussion and slightly mobile. A pulpectomy was carried out before fitting another crown. The left buccal segment continues to be in Class III molar relationship. Figure 8-6 shows the clinical appearance at a review appointment 1 week later.

DISCUSSION

The developmental defects of the enamel index[4] can be used to classify alterations in enamel such as those seen on the present patient's teeth. The non-specificity of appearance of these defects, together with the confounding posteruptive changes (such as caries, attrition, and fracture of enamel) makes etiologic diagnosis problematic.[5] However, regardless of the etiology, in the young child these defects are managed on their merits together with those of the patient.

Clinically, developmental defects of enamel such as those seen in our patient's teeth share many of the characteristics of molar–incisor hypomineralization (MIH). It has been postulated that the increased levels of anxiety and behavioral management problems often noted in children with MIH[6] are related to the early and more frequent dental interventions these children require. However, it has also been shown that bacterial invasion, and subsequently pulpal inflammation, are associated with the more porous enamel found in MIH, and that this may be responsible for both the hypersensitivity the children report, and the difficulty dentists often find in achieving effective local anesthesia.[7] Regardless of the mechanism, the management of these children presents the clinician with significant challenges, and it is crucial that their dental care does not increase any anxiety through overambitious treatment provision. PMCs are recommended for restoring primary molars affected by developmental enamel defects such as enamel hypoplasia.[8] However, placing them conventionally can be demanding for both the child and the clinician, and they are not a popular treatment option for general dental practitioners in the UK.[9]

A recent clinical trial found that Hall crowns could be placed successfully for the majority of children, and were both more acceptable and more effective than conventional restorations placed by general dental practitioners.[2] Use of Hall crowns allowed our patient's hypoplastic and carious primary molars to be successfully managed without the use of dental injections or caries removal, both of which were beyond his ability to accept. In addition, avoiding what he considered to be unpleasant experiences allowed his confidence to be built up to the level where he was able to accept resin fissure sealants on his first permanent molars. It is likely that these positive experiences with dentistry will leave him well prepared to accept local anesthesia and more invasive treatments should they prove necessary in the future.

Hall PMCs have been investigated, and shown to be effective, for the management of carious primary molars where caries has been sealed in and not removed at all.[2] In the case presented here, they have been used as a restoration to provide coverage, relieving pain, and preventing further deterioration of teeth affected by developmental hypoplasia. Such teeth are commonly victim to caries which, together with fracturing of the unstable enamel structure can lead to rapid and unpredictable loss of tooth substance. PMCs are durable restorations. The Hall crown does not rely on chemical adhesion for retention, which is often difficult with these teeth, and because it provides complete coverage, it can help protect the tooth from a caries attack.

Key Message

The Hall technique is a minimally invasive procedure which may be useful in the management of the young child with caries or developmental defects of primary tooth enamel.

REFERENCES

1. Scottish Dental website. The Hall Technique – Manual. Available at: www.scottishdental.org/index.aspx?o=2187&record=31. Accessed 24 March 2009.
2. Innes NPT, Evans DJP, Stirrups DR. The Hall Technique: a randomized controlled clinical trial of a novel method of managing carious primary molars in general dental practice; acceptability of the technique and outcomes at 23 months. BMC Oral Health 2007;7:18. Available at: www.biomedcentral.com/1472-6831/7/18. Accessed 13 March 2009.
3. Scottish Intercollegiate Guidelines Network website. Prevention and Management of Decay in the Pre-school Child: SIGN Guideline 83, 2005. Available at: www.sign.ac.uk/pdf/sign83.pdf. Accessed 13 March 2009.
4. FDI Commission on Oral Health, Research and Epidemiology. A review of the developmental defects of enamel index (DDE index). Int Dent J 1992;42:411–426.
5. Seow WK. Clinical diagnosis of enamel defects: pitfalls and practical guidelines. Int Dent J 1997;47:173–182.
6. Jalevik B, Klingberg GA. Dental treatment, dental fear and behaviour management problems in children with severe enamel hypomineralization of their permanent first molars. Int J Paediatr Dent 2002;12:24–32.
7. Fagrell TG, Lingstrom P, Olsson S, Steiniger F, Noren JG. Bacterial invasion of dentinal tubules beneath apparently intact but hypomineralized enamel in molar teeth with molar incisor hypomineralization. Int J Paediatr Dent 2008;18:333–340.
8. Kindelan SA, Day P, Nichol R, Willmott N, Fayle SA. UK National Clinical Guidelines in Paediatric Dentistry: Stainless steel preformed crowns for primary molars. Int J Paediatr Dent 2008;18(suppl. 1):20–28.
9. Threlfall AG, Pilkington L, Milsom KM, Blinkhorn AS, Tickle M. General dental practitioners' views on the use of stainless steel crowns to restore primary molars. Br Dent J 2005;199:453–455.

9

Potential of Incomplete Caries Excavation to Arrest Active Caries Lesions and to Maintain Pulp Vitality

Jan Kühnisch
Katharina Bücher
Reinhard Hickel

Key words: caries treatment, arresting caries, incomplete caries excavation, maintain pulp vitality

Age category: 4–7 years

Definition
Restoration related to incomplete caries removal: how "clean" must a cavity be before restoration? "The metabolic activity in dental plaque, the biofilm at the tooth surface, is the driving force behind any loss of mineral from the tooth or cavity surface. ... The role of operative dentistry in caries management is to restore the integrity of the tooth surface so that the patient can clean. Thus, the question, 'How clean must a cavity be before restoration?' may be irrelevant. There is little evidence that infected dentine must be removed prior to sealing the tooth" Kidd (2004).[1]

THE PROBLEM

The dental examination of the two 4-year-old patients described here revealed the typical appearance of early childhood caries type 2 according to Wyne[2] in both patients. Although – according to the parents – the dental destruction was currently not causing their children any symptoms or problems, they were naturally interested in the restoration of the carious lesions. Not having had dental treatment before, both children were approachable. The carious teeth were restored stepwise after the patients had been desensitized, bearing in mind their young age. However, rather than dealing with the systematic treatment of two caries-risk patients, this chapter will mainly explain and discuss restrictive/stepwise caries excavation as part of indirect pulp capping in two primary molars.

CASE DESCRIPTION

History

Medical History
ASA I. According to the parents neither of the children had any general disease. During the infant-toddler stage, there had been no abnormalities. Both children were in good general health, and their physical as well as their mental development was normal for their age. No medications were reported. Both patients had received daily prophylactic vitamin D and fluoride supplements (fluoride 0.25 mg tablet) until the age of 2 years, for prevention of rickets and caries. The regional fluoride content in the drinking water was below 0.25 mg/L.

Dental History
The first visit of the two 4-year-old patients to the pediatric unit of Ludwig-Maximilians-University's department of conservative dentistry and periodontology was due to presence of carious lesions, ie, the need to treat them as well as to prevent future problems. No professional dental advice or care had been sought previously.

Oral Hygiene and Nutrition

At the first appointment, the standard of oral hygiene was unsatisfactory in both children. The history revealed irregular tooth cleaning habits, while the parents admitted not assisting/supervising the cleaning in general. By giving the children (and parents) instructions suitable for their age on how to brush their teeth, as well as by encouraging the parents to check the cleaning results and improve them if necessary, the oral hygiene standard was gradually improved. It was recommended to clean the children's teeth at least twice a day with a fluoride children's toothpaste (500 ppm) until they reached the age of 6 years and to change to a junior toothpaste (1000–1500 ppm) thereafter. The parents were also advised to use fluoridated table salt in the preparation of food.

Diet analysis revealed a high intake of cariogenic/erosive drinks throughout the day, eg, iced tea, apple juice, over the past 2 years. Sweets were not consumed frequently.

Examination

The clinical assessment revealed early childhood caries with the primary molars being considerably more affected than the anterior teeth in both children. While the lesions on smooth surfaces already seemed to be arrested, those in the occlusal pits and fissures appeared more active. The status of craniomandibular growth and tooth eruption corresponded to the patients' chronological age; there were no anomalies of tooth position or occlusal disturbances. Likewise, no enamel disturbances were found.

At the initial examination, plaque-induced gingival inflammation was noted. There were no pathologic findings related to the oral mucosa. Compliance was satisfactory for both children at the initial visit, as well as during the clinical examination and the first professional tooth cleaning session.

Additional Investigations

No other investigations were carried out during the initial visits.

TREATMENT AIMS

The following preventive and therapeutic goals were agreed with the parents:

- Introduction of measures to lower the risk of caries substantially in the long term: a tooth-friendly diet, effective daily toothbrushing, and adequate fluoride usage.
- 'Easy' – less invasive – activities such as cleaning the children's teeth with a rotating bristle brush and the placing of sealants over non-cavitated pits and fissures. These were intended to promote systematic familiarization of the young patients with dental treatment. After successful desensitization, the overall restorative treatment was scheduled.
- According to the traditional approach of restorative treatment, two deep caries lesions (in the mandibular left primary second molar (75; case 1) and in the mandibular right primary second molar (85; case 2) would have been excavated and filled with an adhesive restoration. However, due to the limited compliance of the patients it was decided to modify the treatment by removing the biofilm and the majority of the destroyed tissue and leaving the infected dentin.

TREATMENT OPTIONS

Definitive

With practice of the preventive measures and systematic desensitization, the children grew more accepting of dental treatment. Since it had been impossible to remove the carious lesions fully and to carry out all the necessary steps for the placement of adhesive fillings as a result of the children's refusal to cooperate, their teeth were monitored via patient recall. Permanent adhesive restorations were planned either when patient compliance had significantly improved or when the temporary filling failed.

Alternatives

Full restorative treatment would probably have resulted in pulpal perforation in both teeth during traditional excavation procedures. The ensuing endodontic treatment – most likely pulpotomy – was considered as being too complex for the children.

Rationale

Dental treatment of patients with early childhood caries is often carried out under conscious sedation or general anesthesia because of the negative restoration–compliance balance of the child. As children become older, their willingness to cooperate generally increases and can also be improved by using behavioral management techniques. Beside efforts to treat small children without the use of conscious sedation or general anesthesia, recent discussions have focused on how to deal with deep dentin carious lesions in symptomless teeth. As complete excavation often leaves the pulp exposed, some authors have advocated a minimally invasive approach.[1,3,4] According to them the removal of the biofilm and the sealing of the cavity have a major role in the attempt to arrest the carious process. This approach could help the pediatric dentist be more restrictive in using conscious sedation and/or general anesthesia on the one hand and avoid pulp exposure on the other hand.

TREATMENT AND FOLLOW-UP

CASE 1

Treatment

The active deep occlusal lesion in the mandibular left primary second molar (75) was treated during the third appointment. As a result of the patient's reduced compliance the caries tissue could not be removed completely as intended. Treatment therefore consisted of incomplete excavation of the demineralized dentin, application of calcium hydroxide and sealing the tooth with a glass-ionomer cement. The parents were informed about the clinical status and told to return if the restoration failed or the child felt pain. During the following sessions – with improved patient compliance – the remaining fillings were placed.

Posttreatment Evaluation/Follow-up

After the initial treatment at the age of 4, the patient attended follow-up appointments at regular intervals. One year after treatment, clinical examination of the mandibular left primary second molar (75) revealed no pathologic findings. The tooth was symptomless and reacted positively to a vitality test with a cold stimulus. The filling was also fully intact (Fig. 9-1). In addition to the clinical examination, bilateral bitewing radiographs were taken for caries detection/diagnosis (Fig. 9-2). While the deep lesion on the mandibular left primary first molar (74) was restored promptly after detection, the intact restoration in the mandibular left primary second molar (75) was further monitored. During the initial treatment of the then 4-year-old patient, it was not possible to excavate the demineralized dentin completely as a result of the child's limited compliance.

At the age of 6 years, when the patient was fully compliant, it was decided to replace the occlusal filling in the mandibular left primary second molar (75) (Fig. 9-3). Figure 9-4 shows the clinical appearance of the arrested residual carious lesion and the restoration procedure. Figures 9-5 to 9-7 show the clinical appearance of the tooth during the 3-year follow-up period.

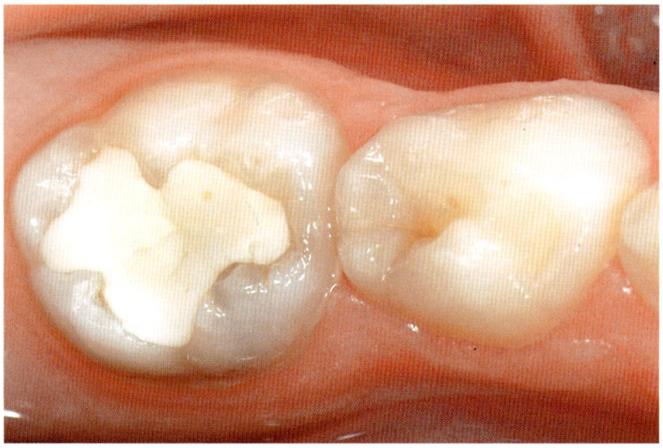

Fig. 9-1 Clinical situation of the symptomless lower left primary molars at the age of 5, and a glass-ionomer cement restoration in the mandibular left primary second molar (75).

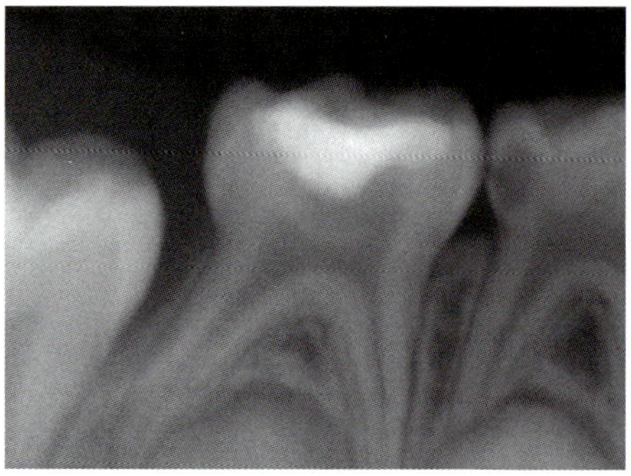

Fig. 9-2 The left bitewing radiograph shows a D4 lesion on the distal surface of the mandibular left primary first molar (74) and a residual caries lesion beneath the pulp under the restoration in the mandibular left primary second molar (75).

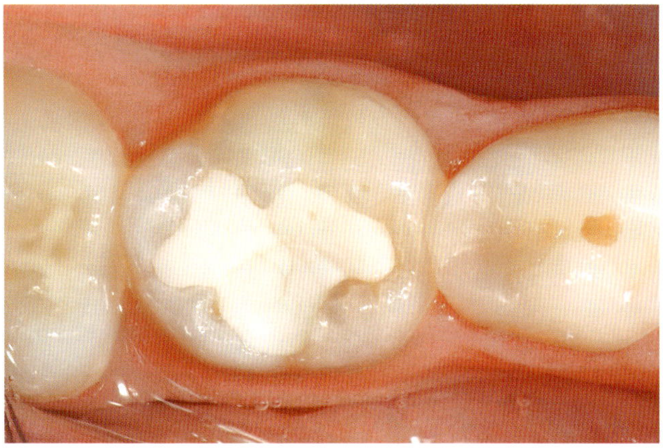

Fig. 9-3 Two-year follow-up: following substantial improvements in patient compliance, re-treatment of the mandibular left primary second molar (75) was scheduled after observing signs of functional restoration failure (small hairline cracks, imperfect marginal integrity) 2 years after the initial restoration had been placed and because of the inferior long-term prognosis of glass-ionomer cement. Both the molars had not caused any pain in the previous 2 years and reacted promptly to a cold stimulus.

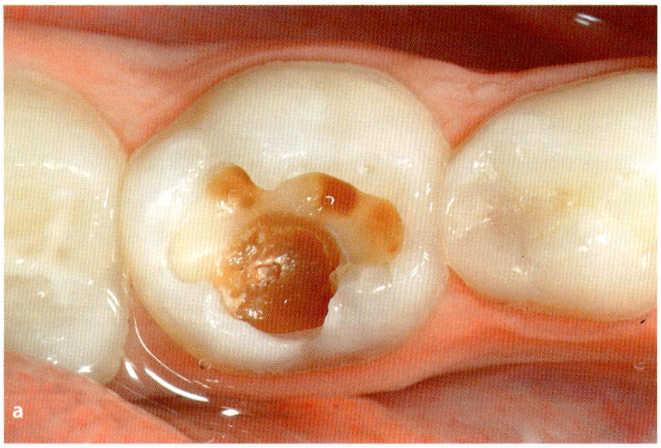

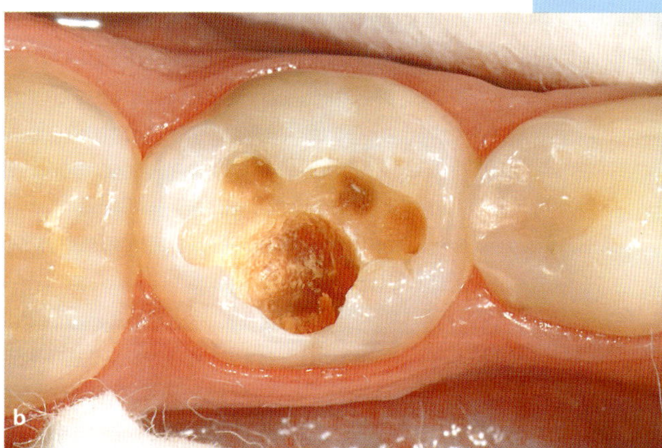

Fig. 9-4a Re-treatment after 2 years: on removal of the calcium hydroxide base quite wet, leathery, and discolored dentin was detected. The caries process was arrested.

Fig. 9-4b The leathery dentin was excavated and the final cavity floor showed dry, solid, and discolored dentin. The peripheral cavity margins were cleaned as carefully as possible to ensure excellent marginal adaptation of the adhesive restoration.

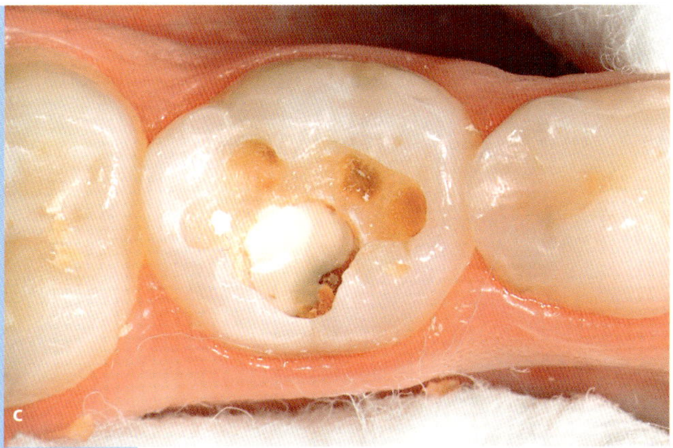

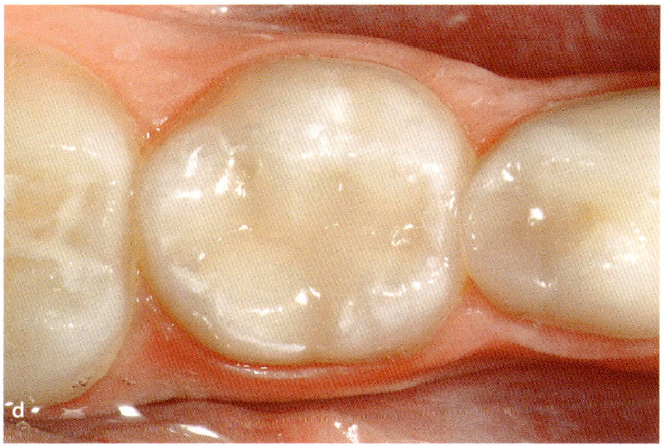

Fig. 9-4c Calcium hydroxide base was placed on the cavity floor.

Fig. 9-4d The resin composite was placed after conventional etching (~10 seconds) and application of a light-curing dentin/enamel bonding agent.

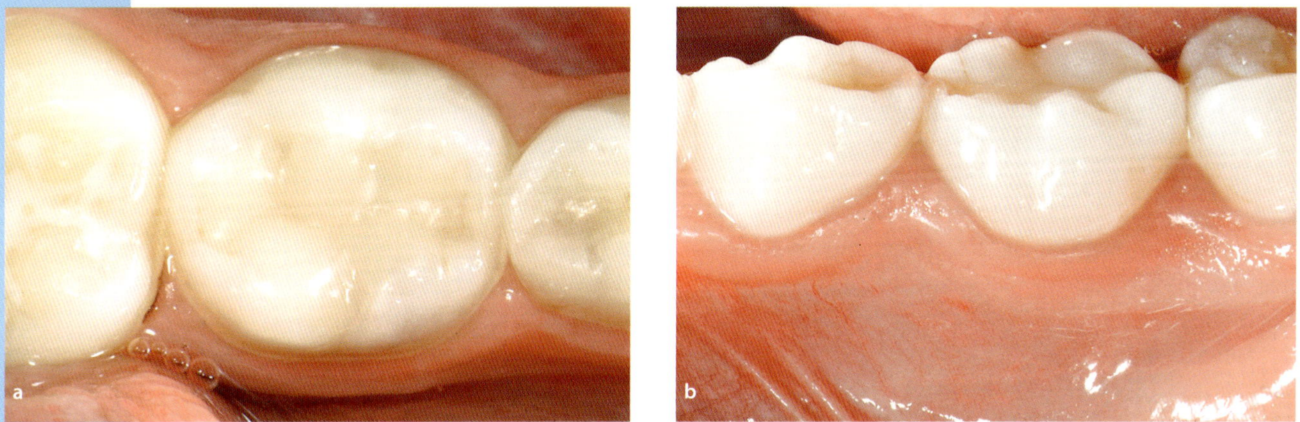

Fig. 9-5a,b One-year follow-up of the definitive restoration showed that it was both functionally and esthetically satisfactory. Both the molars (74, 75) were symptomless and vital. No apical inflammation was detected.

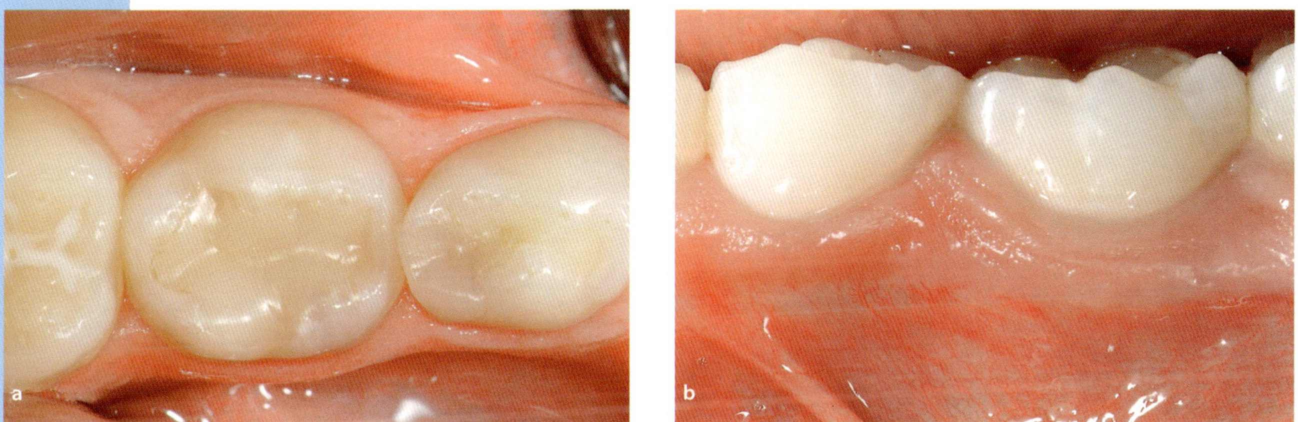

Fig. 9-6a,b Two-year follow-up of the composite restoration in tooth 75 indicated no functional or esthetical failure; both primary molars were symptomless and vital. No apical inflammations were detectable.

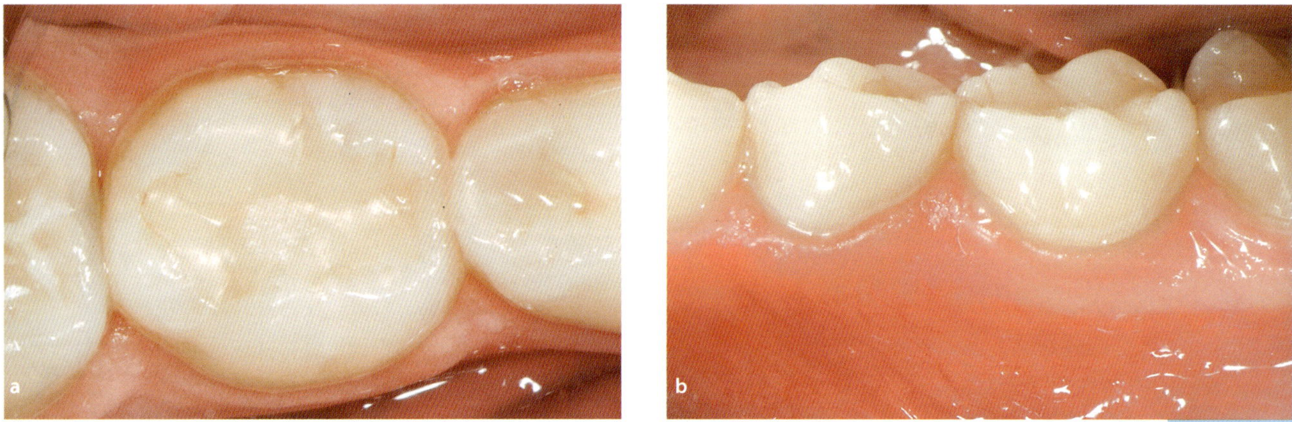

Fig. 9-7a,b Three-year follow-up of the definitive restorations – 5 years after the beginning of the treatment – underlined the successful treatment strategy for both primary molars. The restorations were completely retained, with no fracture lines, cracks, or marginal gaps. Both teeth were symptomless and vital, with no evidence of inflammation, eg, fistula, swelling.

CASE 2

Treatment

After the patient's first visit, professional tooth cleaning, pit and fissure sealing, and easily applicable fillings were carried out for slow, gradual exposure. The active occlusal lesion of the symptomless mandibular second primary molar (85) was excavated during the fourth session (Fig. 9-8a). Due to the girl's insufficient compliance it was impossible to remove the carious process completely, and the remaining soft, wet and brown discolored dentin (Fig. 9-8b) was capped with a calcium hydroxide suspension. Additionally, a calcium hydroxide liner was placed to protect and stabilize the aqueous suspension. The cavity was sealed with a self-etching bonding agent and filled with a composite material (Fig. 9-8c). The parents were informed about the incomplete caries removal as well as the prospect of replacing the restoration later on.

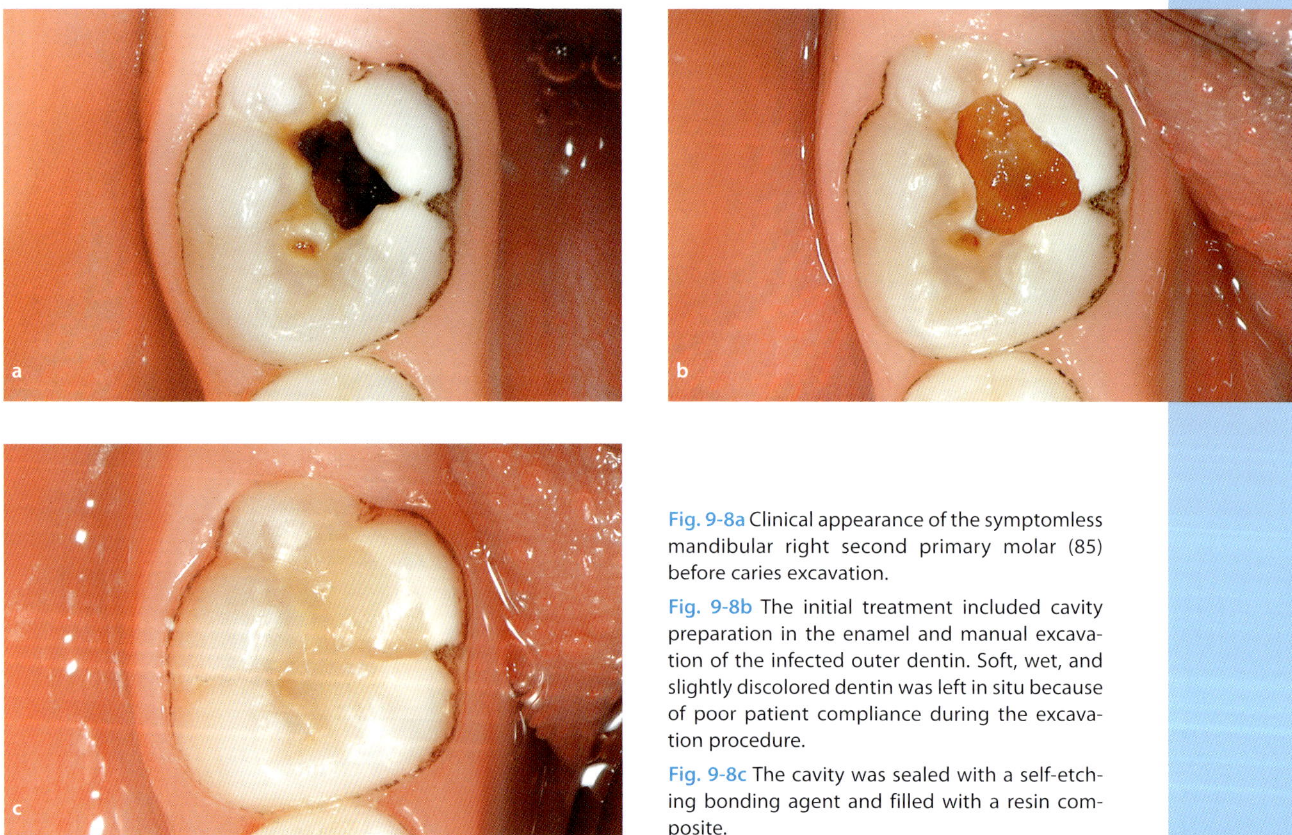

Fig. 9-8a Clinical appearance of the symptomless mandibular right second primary molar (85) before caries excavation.

Fig. 9-8b The initial treatment included cavity preparation in the enamel and manual excavation of the infected outer dentin. Soft, wet, and slightly discolored dentin was left in situ because of poor patient compliance during the excavation procedure.

Fig. 9-8c The cavity was sealed with a self-etching bonding agent and filled with a resin composite.

Posttreatment Evaluation/Follow-up

As patient compliance steadily improved from one appointment to next, the range of dental care options increased. One year after treatment had started – at the age of 5 – bilateral bitewing radiographs were taken to check for approximal caries lesions (Figs 9-9a, 9-9b) but no lesions were found. Clinically, the mandibular right primary second molar was symptomless and the occlusal restoration was intact. However, the bitewing radiograph illustrated extension of the residual caries. Two years after treatment had started it was decided to replace the fillings due to insufficient margins (Fig. 9-10, Figs 9-11a to 9-11d). One year after re-treatment, the tooth was symptomless and vital, and the definitive restoration was fully intact (Fig. 9-12).

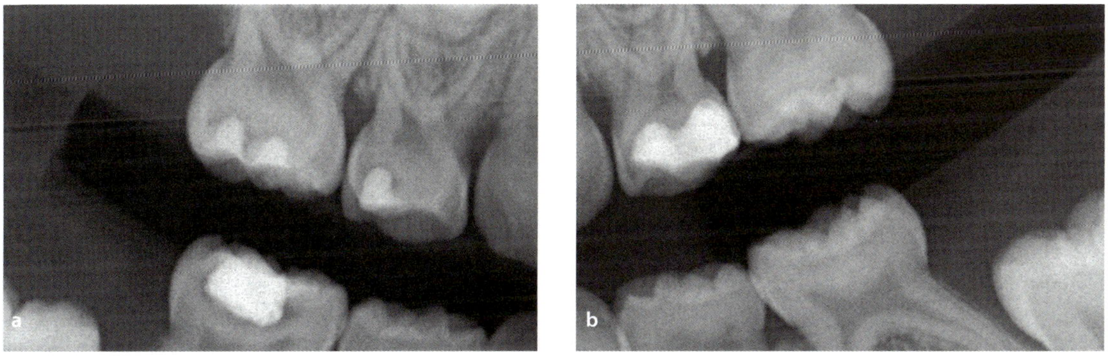

Fig. 9-9a,b Bilateral bitewing radiographs were taken 1 year after finishing the initial treatment, mainly to investigate the proximal surfaces. Residual caries was detected in both maxillary primary first molars (64, 65) and the mandibular right second primary molar (85). The superficial, non-cavitated occlusal dentin lesions in the maxillary left primary second molar (65) and mandibular left primary second molar (75) were sealed during the initial treatment.

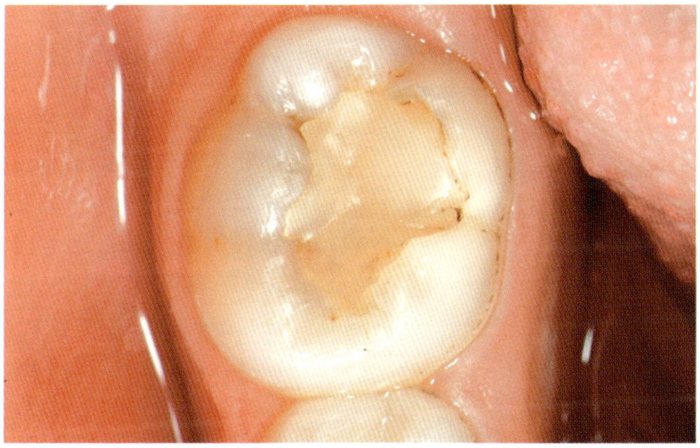

Fig. 9-10 Clinical appearance of the occlusal composite filling after two years. Due to lack of marginal integrity and the associated risk of bacterial leakage it was decided to replace the restoration. At the age of 6 and after regular preventive treatment, the patient is now fully cooperative.

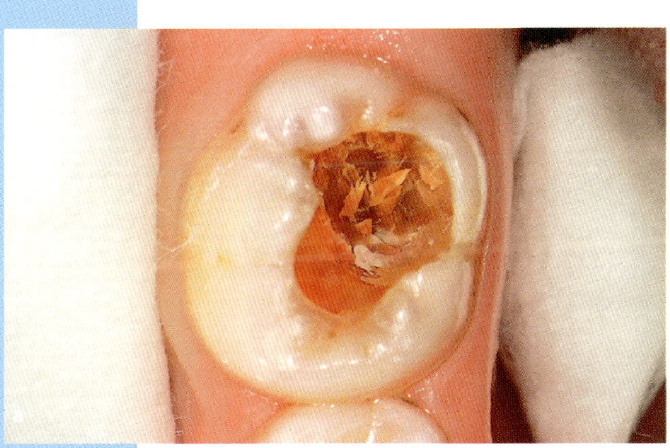

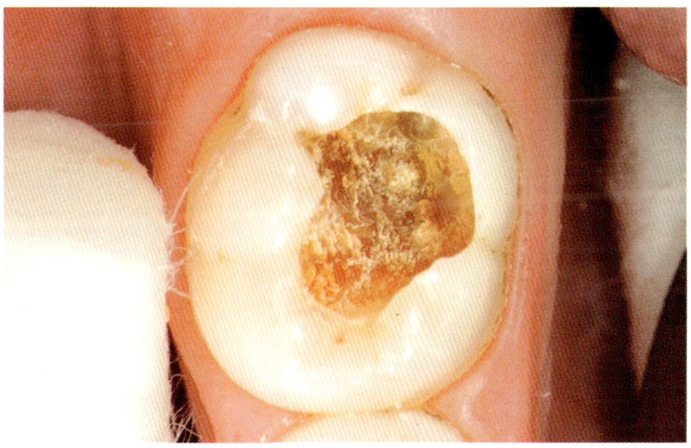

Fig. 9-11a Re-treatment after two years. The soft, wet, and discolored dentin that had previously been left behind was now an arrested lesion. The dentin appeared to be dry, leathery, and discolored.

Fig. 9-11b The leathery dentin was manually excavated and the final cavity floor showed dry, solid, and discolored dentin. All peripheral enamel and dentin margins were cleaned as carefully as possible to guarantee excellent marginal adaptation of the adhesive restoration.

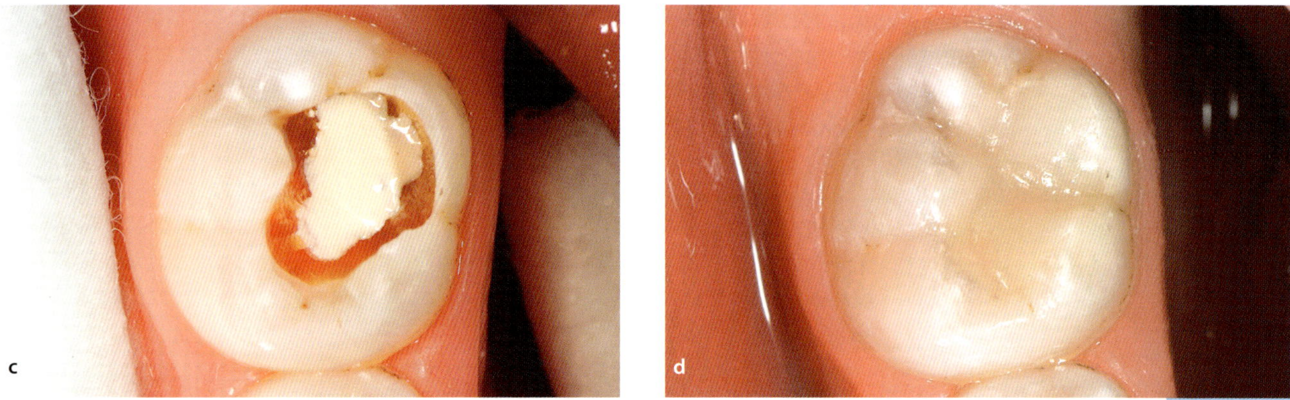

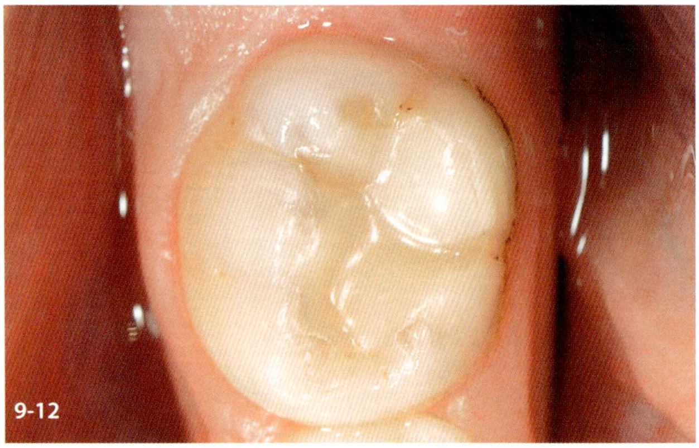

Fig. 9-11c Calcium hydroxide liner was placed on the cavity floor.

Fig. 9-11d After etching (~10 seconds) and application of the bonding resin (light-curing dentin/enamel bonding agent), the cavity was filled with a resin composite.

Fig. 9-12 One-year follow-up of the restoration showed no functional failure of the restoration. The tooth was symptomless and vital.

DISCUSSION

In the two cases described in this chapter, the initial treatment goal – complete caries excavation – had to be modified as a result of the young patients' limited compliance. The carious tissue was only partly removed and an easy-to-apply temporary filling was placed, thus maintaining the patients' compliance as well as avoiding pulp therapy. As the cavities were limited to the occlusal surface in both children, this meant better prognosis than if the cavities had involved several tooth surfaces or had margins extended into dentin. Frequent follow-up checks are considered essential to detect inadequate fillings early to help prevent bacterial microleakage as well as reinfection of the previous active lesion.

The results of the long-term follow-up show the potential of indirect pulp treatment for primary teeth, and also support the theory that the treatment can be successful even though softened dentin remains while the cavity is sealed definitely.[1] This demonstrates that, in particular cases, a more conservative approach can be used for caries excavation. Supporters of this approach refer to the lower pulp exposure risk[5,6] and the arrest of the carious lesion[7] as major benefits. The arrested lesion encourages the obliteration of the dentinal tubules as well as the formation of reactionary dentin, thus reducing the permeability of the remaining dentin. The apparent irrelevance of the infected dentin after sealing the cavity is biologically logical if it is accepted that the caries process is driven by the biofilm and its reflection is the lesion in the dental hard tissues.[1] Clinical and radiographic[8] success rates of 90% – over a study period of 4 years – as well as histologic success rates of >70%[9] provide evidence that this treatment of deep caries lesions is a promising approach in primary teeth.

Key Message
As long as the cavity is sealed completely and checkups made regularly, even incomplete caries excavation may be considered a possible treatment option for primary teeth.

REFERENCES

1. Kidd EAM. How 'clean' must a cavity be before restoration? Caries Res 2004;38:305–313.
2. Wyne AH. Early childhood caries: nomenclature and case definition. Community Dent Oral Epidemiol 1999;27:313–315.
3. Ricketts DNJ, Kidd EAM, Innes N, Clarkson J. Complete or ultraconservative removal of decayed tissue in unfilled teeth (Cochrane review). In: The Cochrane Library, 2006:Issue 4. Chichester: Wiley.
4. Rodd HD, Waterhouse PJ, Fuks AB, Fayle SA, Moffat MA. UK national clinical guidelines in paediatric dentistry: pulp therapy for primary molars. Int J Paediatr Dent 2006;16(suppl. 1):15–23.
5. Magnusson BO, Sundell SO. Stepwise excavation of deep carious lesions in primary molars. J Int Ass Dent Child 1977;8:36–40.
6. Leskell E, Ridell K, Cvek M, Mejare I. Pulp exposure after stepwise versus direct complete excavation of deep carious lesions in young posterior permanent teeth. Endod Dent Traumatol 1996;12:192–196.
7. Mertz-Fairhurst EJ, Curtis JW Jr, Ergle JW, Rueggeberg FA, Adair SM. Ultraconservative and cariostatic sealed restorations: results at year 10. J Am Dent Assoc 1998;129:55–66.
8. Marchi JJ, de Araujo FB, Fröner AM, Straffon LH, Nör JE. Indirect pulp capping in the primary dentition: a 4 year follow-up study. J Clin Pediatr Dent 2006;31:68–71.
9. Heinrich R, Kneist S, Künzel W. Klinisch-kontrollierte Untersuchung zur Caries-profunda-Therapie. Dtsch Zahnärztl Z 1991;46:581–584.

10 Management of Sequelae in the Permanent Incisors After Trauma in the Primary Dentition

Frèdèric Obry
Rèmy Mathis
Marie-Cècile Manière

Key words: dental trauma, developmental disturbances, forced eruption

Age category: 7 12 years

Definition
A sequela is a pathologic condition that develops as a result of a prior disease, injury, or attack. Impaction is defined as the total or partial lack of eruption of a tooth after the normal age of eruption. If the third molars are not considered, the maxillary canines and the central incisors are the teeth most likely to remain impacted. One of the common causes is trauma in primary dentition. Clinically, impaction is associated with esthetic and functional consequences.

THE PROBLEM

Susie, a 7½-year-old girl, was referred by her dentist to the pediatric dentistry department for delayed eruption of a central incisor.

CASE DESCRIPTION

History

Medical History
ASA I. Susie's medical history was unremarkable with no systemic contraindications to surgery or orthodontic treatment.

Dental History
Susie experienced trauma to the maxillary anterior region at the age of 23 months, with intrusion of the left primary maxillary central incisor (61). The mother stated that this primary incisor had re-erupted spontaneously within approximately 3 months, and exfoliated at the age of 6½, at the same time as the right maxillary primary central incisor.

Oral Hygiene
At the initial examination, oral hygiene was poor. Susie and her parents were given instructions to help improve her oral hygiene.

Examination

On clinical examination, the upper left central permanent incisor (21) was unerupted whereas the right central incisor was present in a normal position within the dental arch (Fig. 10-1). The left maxillary lateral incisor (22) had also erupted, and was rotated, partially closing the space for the left central incisor.

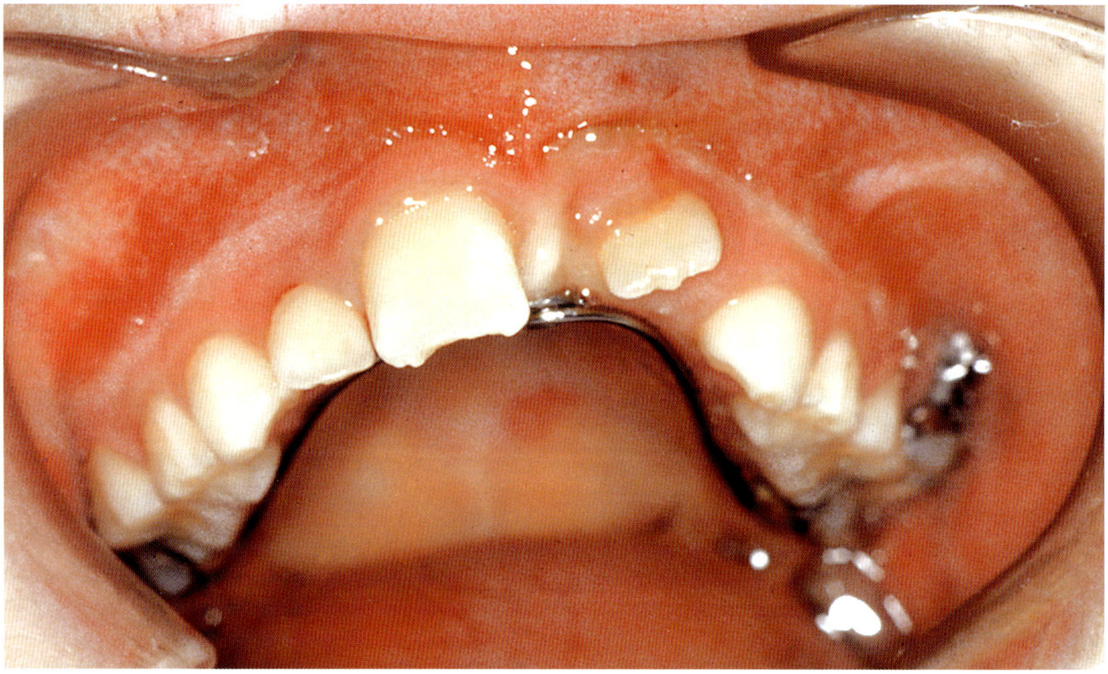

Fig. 10-1 Intraoral view of missing left maxillary central incisor (21) in a 7½-year-old girl. The right maxillary permanent central incisor and the left maxillary permanent lateral incisor are present. Note the rotation of the left maxillary lateral incisor and the space closure.

Additional Investigations

On the occlusal radiograph, the maxillary left permanent central incisor (21) was impacted. Incomplete root development and open apices of the central incisors were observed (Fig. 10-2).

The exact position of the tooth was determined by computed tomography. The axial reconstruction showed the degree of dilaceration of the maxillary left central incisor (21) (Fig. 10-3a). Three-dimensional reconstruction confirmed the high position of this tooth with the crown being horizontal and adjacent to the anterior nasal spine (Fig. 10-3b).

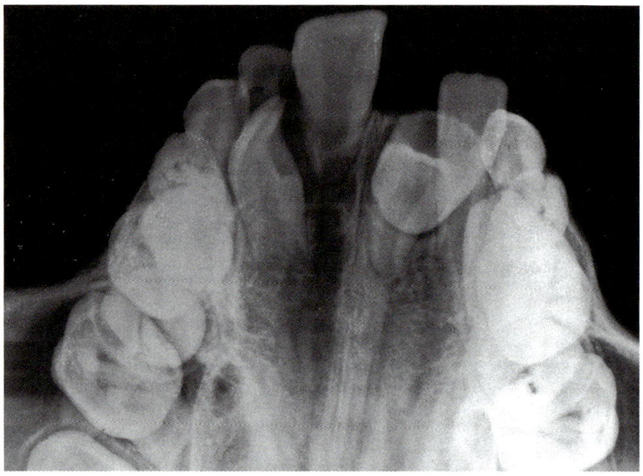

Fig. 10-2 Occlusal radiograph at the initial examination showing impaction and displacement of the left permanent maxillary central incisor (21), which has an open apex.

TREATMENT OPTIONS

Definitive

The therapeutic modality chosen was surgical exposure and orthodontic traction to force eruption of the maxillary permanent left central incisor (21).

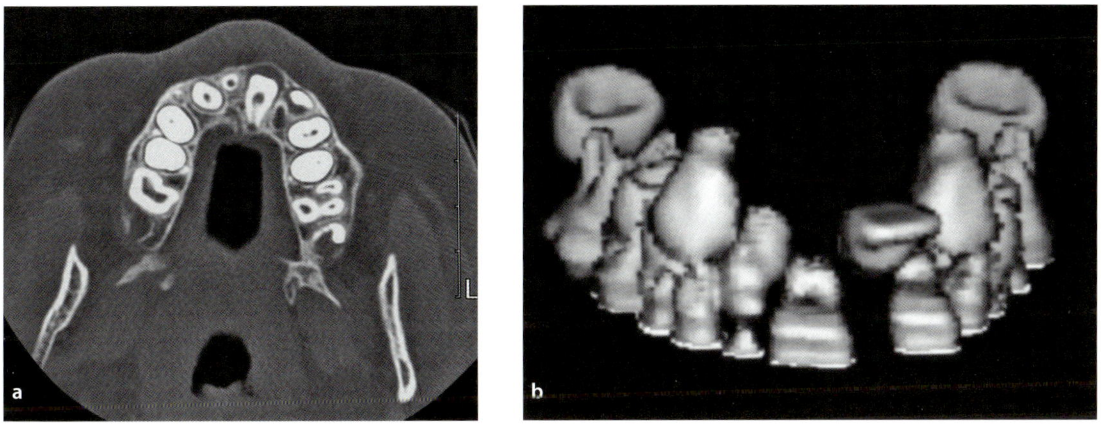

Fig. 10-3a,b Computed tomography: Fig. 10-3a axial reconstruction showing the exact position of the maxillary left central incisor (21) and root development; Fig. 10-3b Three-dimensional reconstruction shows slight crown–root angulation of 21.

Alternatives

Other treatment options were discussed and included:

- extraction of the impacted maxillary left central incisor (21) followed by conventional prosthesis and implant placement at the end of the growth period
- extraction of the maxillary left central incisor (21) followed by autogenous tooth transplantation.

These options were considered to be unfavorable because of the age of the patient and the negative esthetic impact.

TREATMENT AND FOLLOW-UP

Treatment

Prior to the surgery, the parents were informed about the possible risks of the chosen treatment, and Susie was given additional oral hygiene instructions. Adequate space was regained by orthodontic treatment with an appliance consisting of a transpalatal bar cemented on the first permanent upper molars and used as anchorage for extruding the maxillary left central incisor (21) (Fig. 10-4). Surgical crown exposure was performed under local anesthesia (Fig. 10-5). After bonding a

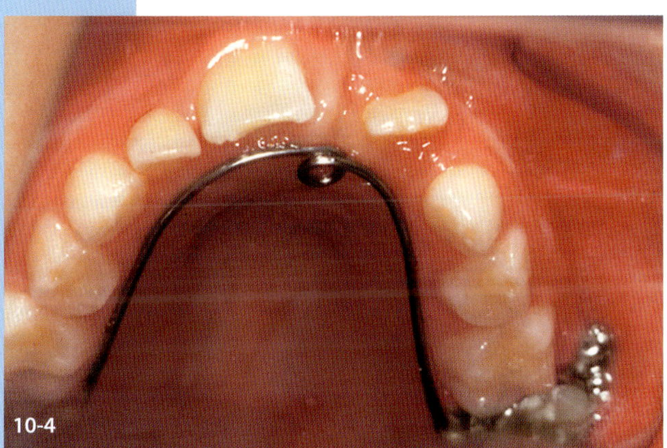

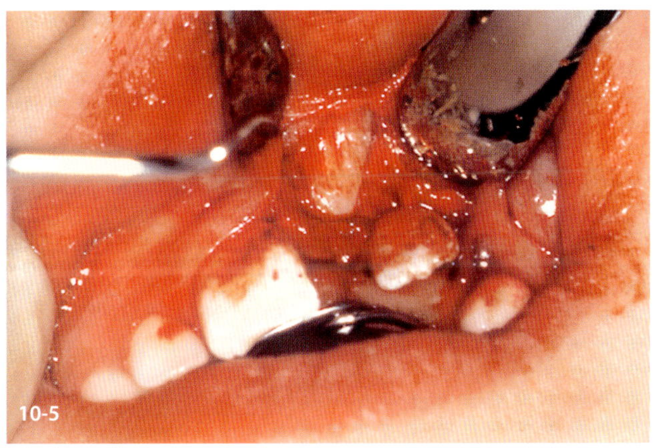

Fig. 10-4 Orthodontic appliance to regain adequate space.

Fig. 10-5 First surgical intervention. Exposure of the palatal surface of the maxillary left central incisor (21).

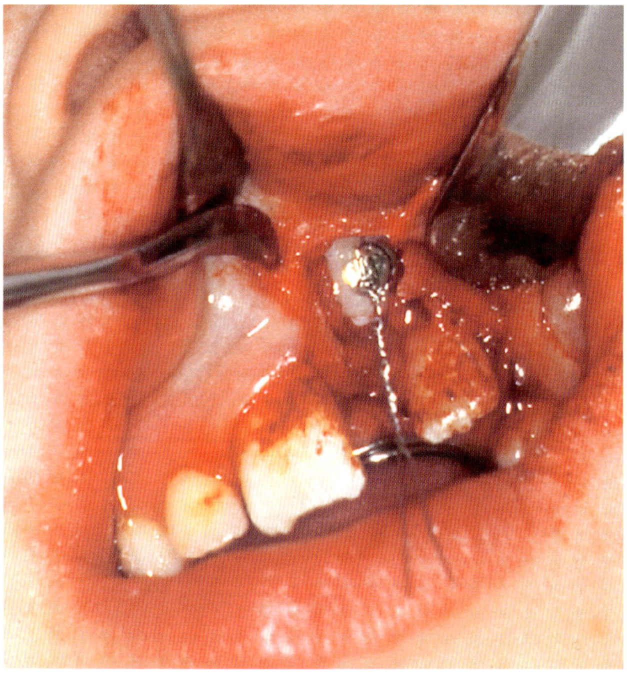

Fig. 10-6 Lingual button bonded on the palatal surface of the impacted incisor.

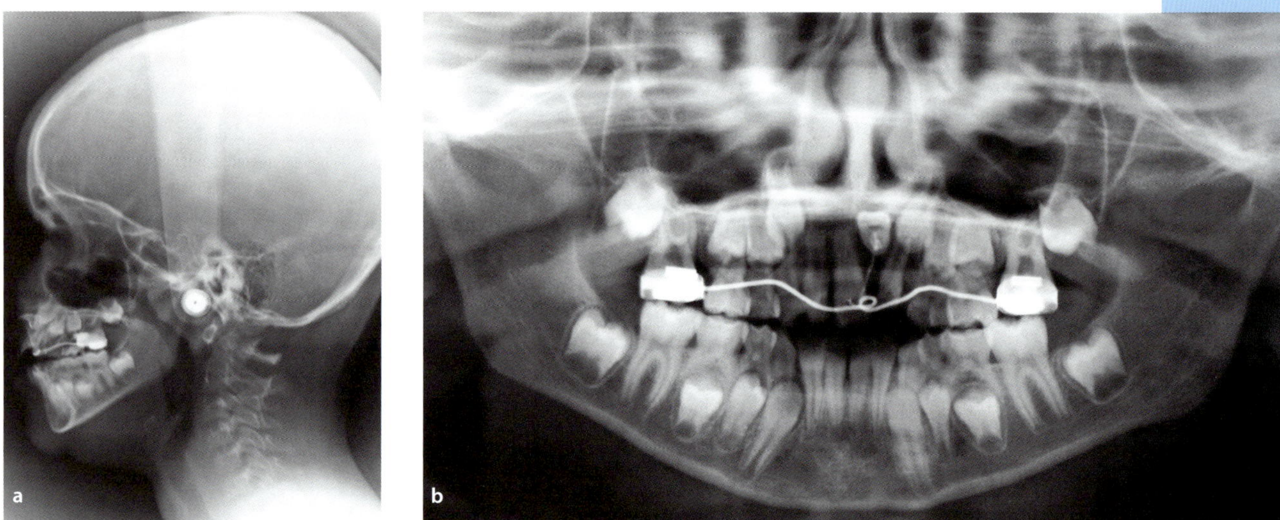

Fig. 10-7a,b Radiographs showing the placement of the fixed appliance and initial tooth movement.

button on the palatal surface of the impacted tooth, a gentle force was applied with an elastic thread tied to the palatal bar (Fig. 10-6, Figs 10-7a, 10-7b). Following extrusion, the tooth was moved into its usual position in the maxillary arch with conventional orthodontic treatment. Eruption was periodically monitored, and the complete eruption and positioning were achieved in 24 months.

Key Message

Forced eruption and orthodontic alignment of an impacted incisor can help achieve a complete dental arch with a stable occlusion, healthy periodontal status, and good esthetics. The successful repositioning of the impacted tooth depends on several factors, such as initial position of the tooth, stage of tooth formation, root morphology and angulation, appropriate bone removal during the surgical procedure, the patient's age and level of cooperation. The use of gentle orthodontic forces to move the tooth gradually prevents bracket debonding, ankylosis, and gingival loss.

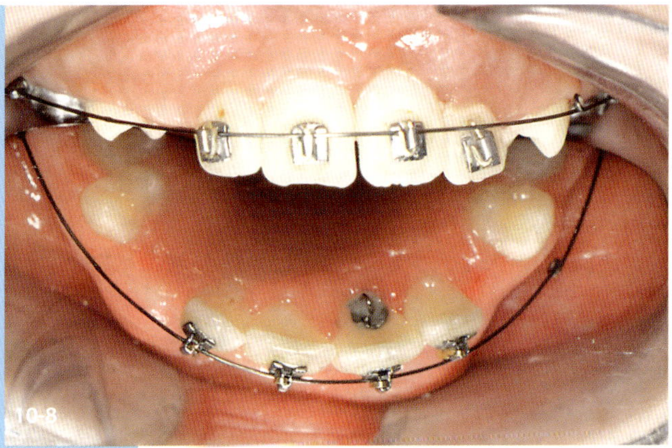

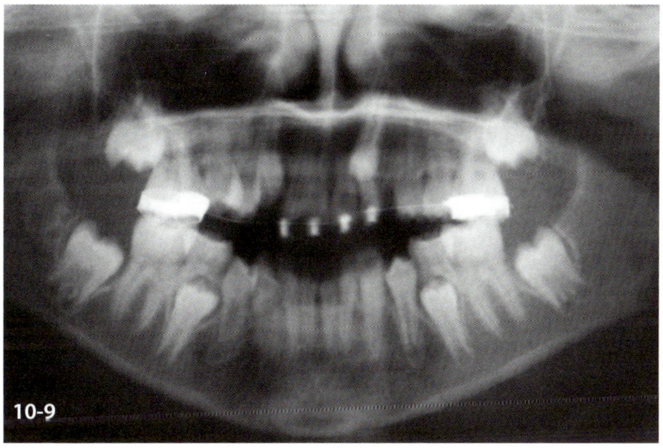

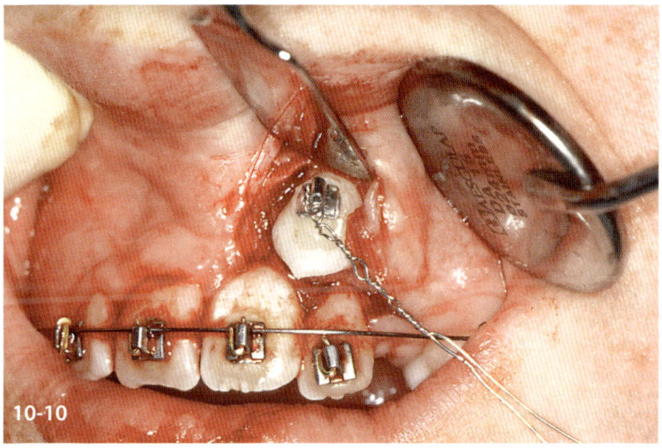

Fig. 10-8 Conventional orthodontic treatment after 2 years.

Fig. 10-9 Panoramic radiographs 2 years after treatment. Note the ectopic position of the maxillary left canine (23).

Fig. 10-10 Second surgical intervention to expose the buccal surface of the maxillary left canine (23) and bonding of orthodontic attachment.

Posttreatment Evaluation/Follow-up

Following orthodontic traction, the tooth was clinically healthy and functioned adequately (Fig. 10-8, Fig. 10-9). The attached gingiva and periodontium were healthy.

The traction of the impacted central incisor may have induced a distal displacement of the axis of the lateral incisor, preventing the normal eruption of the adjacent canine, which was now impacted. Thus, at the age of 11 years, Susie underwent surgical exposure of the impacted left maxillary canine (23), followed by orthodontic repositioning without extraction of the maxillary left first premolar (24) (Fig. 10-10). The final positioning of the canine was achieved in 12 months. A small degree of root resorption was detectable in all the incisors, but there were no carious lesions.

Key Message

Regular clinical and radiographic follow-up after trauma in primary teeth is important, as it allows early detection of sequelae in the permanent teeth, such as a dilacerated and impacted incisor.

Twelve years after the initial examination (patient's age: 20 years), the maxillary left central incisor was stable and exhibited normal sound on percussion (no ankylosis). The panoramic radiograph revealed obliteration of the root canal and pronounced resorption of the root, which was shorter compared with the roots of the other incisors. The pulp canal obliteration may have been caused by the orthodontic traction. Eight years after the end of the active orthodontic treatment, the apical resorption was severe, with a root length of 10 mm (Fig. 10-11). There was no increased mobility of the maxillary left central incisor (21) compared with the adjacent teeth. The apical root resorption which was detected during the follow-up in all permanent maxillary incisors may have been related to the orthodontic traction of the impacted canine.

After two successive surgical procedures in the anterior maxilla, the alveolar bone height of the exposed incisor and canine was good and adequate function had been obtained. The attached gin-

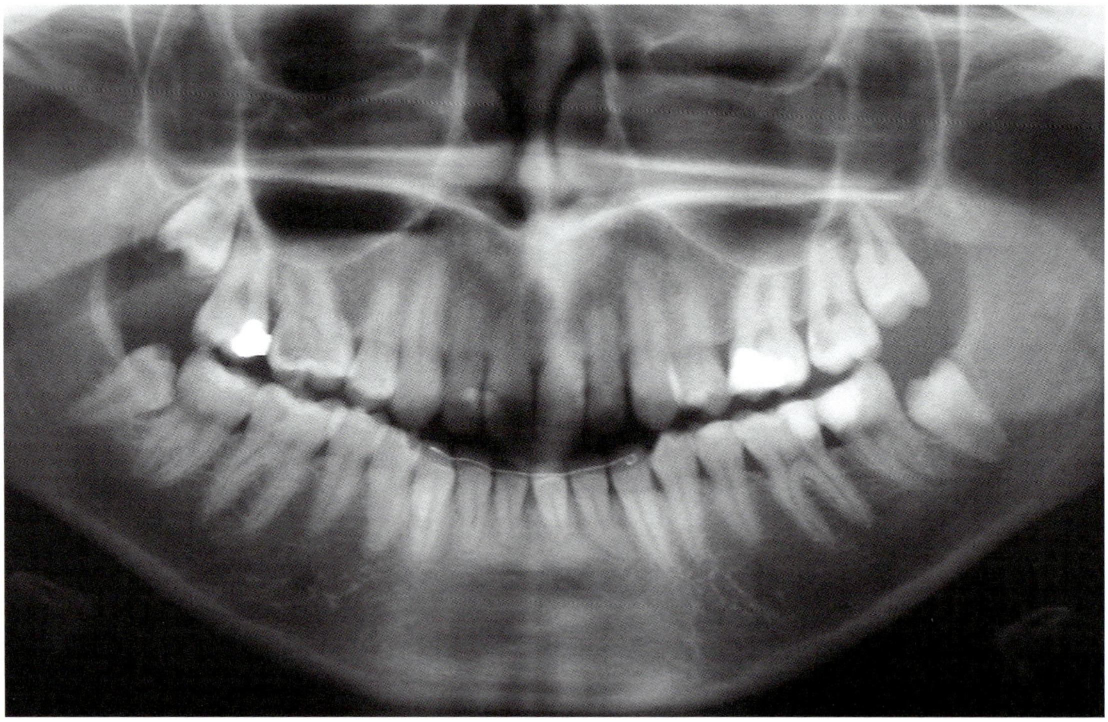

Fig. 10-11 Panoramic radiograph 12 years after the beginning of treatment, showing resorption of the incisor roots and root canal obliteration in the maxillary left central incisor (21).

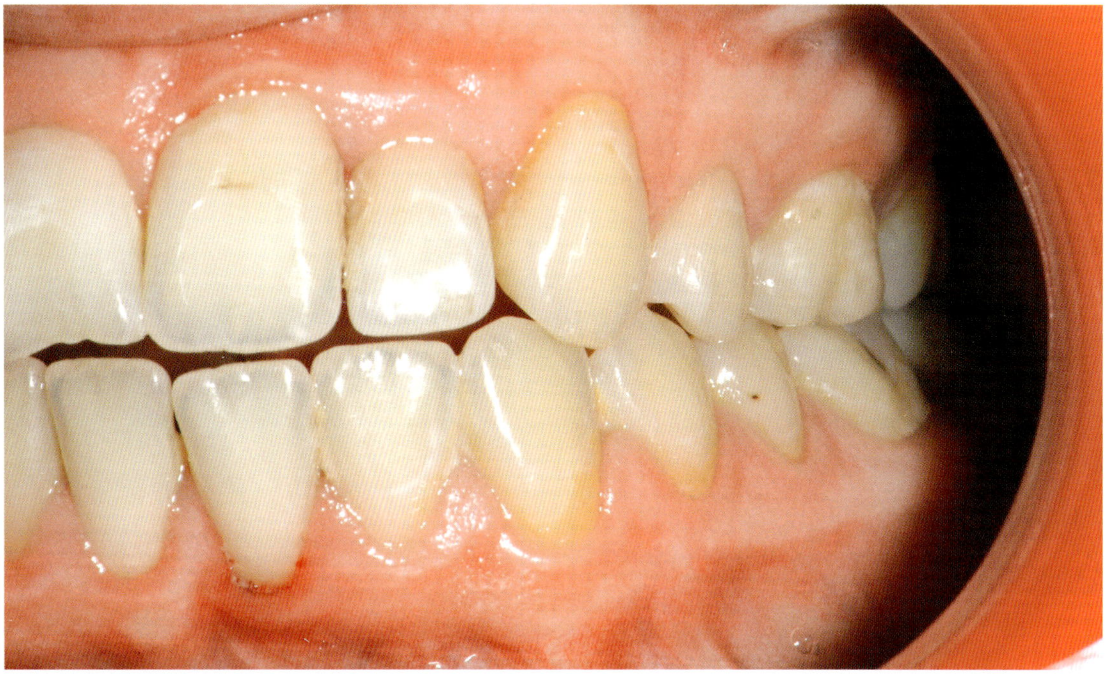

Fig. 10-12 Intraoral appearance after 12 years.

giva was in good health, despite a difference in the level of the gingival contour between the two central incisors, providing an esthetically acceptable appearance. No discoloration of the crown was observed. Nevertheless, poor oral hygiene of this young adult patient could compromise the final result (Fig. 10-12). Increased caries activity was also noticed and it was noted that the patient worked in a sweetshop. Thus, the very long-term prognosis is uncertain as increased mobility could be expected if the periodontium will not remain healthy.

DISCUSSION

Trauma to the primary dentition may cause developmental disturbances in the permanent dentition, which can be encountered in the coronal (enamel hypoplasia, crown dilaceration) as well as in the root region (dilaceration, partial or complete arrest of root formation). The sequelae affecting the whole permanent tooth germ range from delayed eruption to severe sequestration of the developing tooth germ and other types of malformation such as odontoma.[1] In the case of an impacted incisor, the clinical consequences in a young patient could be esthetic, occlusal, functional, and phonetic.[2]

Intrusive injuries of primary incisors are associated with a high risk of sequelae in the successor teeth. The age of the child at the time of injury, the direction and severity of the intrusion, and the presence of alveolar bone fractures are the main variables influencing the effect of primary tooth intrusion on the permanent tooth germs. The highest incidence of this type of trauma occurs between the ages of 1 and 3 years.[3]

The clinical consequences of impaction associated with crown or root dilaceration are esthetic and functional. In most cases, a single tooth is impacted. Forced eruption of the impacted tooth seems to be the most favorable therapeutic option.[4,5] Nevertheless, little is known about the long-term prognosis of impacted dilacerated incisors after surgical exposure and orthodontic traction. Careful assessment of an impacted incisor is required to choose the best surgical approach. Thus, complementing the conventional radiographs with a computed tomography scan is useful to assess precisely the morphology of the tooth as well as its position.[6]

The etiology of canine impaction is different from impaction of incisors. The causes are multifactorial but mainly local, such as the long path of eruption, discrepancies in tooth size–arch length ratio, presence of odontoma or supernumerary teeth, and also history of local trauma.

In various studies, the risk of orthodontically induced root resorption has been correlated with dental anomalies such as taurodontism, invagination, agenesis, ectopic eruption, and supernumerary or atypical teeth. Traumatic factors also have a role in the etiology of resorption. Orthodontic forces may be responsible for this phenomenon. A large majority of authors confirm that a positive correlation exists between the type and magnitude of the orthodontic force, the length of treatment, and the existence and severity of root resorption.[7]

In the present case, two consecutive orthodontic treatments were performed, in the context of developmental anomalies, resulting in an increased risk of root resorption. Another etiologic factor may have been the inherent pressure on the incisors of the ectopically positioned canine.

In case of root resorption, careful clinical and intraoral radiographic supervision is recommended on a long-term basis. As plaque-induced gingivitis may increase the risk of tooth mobility in the case of severe root resorption, oral hygiene has to be regularly evaluated and reinforced.[8]

Surgical exposure followed by orthodontic repositioning is a clinical challenge as the compliance of the child is required for a long procedure to move the tooth into its proper position.[9] Also, root formation could be abnormal and require endodontic assessment.[10] In conclusion, compared with the prosthetic treatment option, this therapeutic solution is more biocompatible as it preserves the patient's tooth and the bone volume.

Key Message

The long-term viability of impacted incisors after repositioning is generally good. The initial traumatic intrusion of primary incisors as well as the orthodontic traction of an impacted incisor may have also consequences for the development and eruption of the ipsilateral canine. Close and long-term monitoring and multidisciplinary collaboration during the different steps of the treatment are necessary.

REFERENCES

1. Arenas M, Barberia E, Lucavechi T, Maroto M. Severe trauma in the primary dentition – diagnosis and treatment of sequelae in permanent dentition. Dent Traumatol 2006;22:226–230.
2. Diab M, el Badrawy HE. Intrusion injuries of primary incisors. Part III: effects on the permanent successors. Quintessence Int 2000;31:377–384.
3. Andreasen JO. Injuries to developing teeth. In: Andreasen JO, Andreasen FM (eds) Textbook and Color Atlas of Traumatic Injuries to the Teeth. Copenhagen: Mosby, 1994:457–494.
4. Macias E, de Carlos F, Cobo J. Posttraumatic impaction of both maxillary central incisors. Am J Orthod Dentofacial Orthop 2003;124:331–338.
5. Bayram M, Ozer M, Sener I. Maxillary canine impactions related to impacted central incisors: two case reports. J Contemp Dent Pract 2007;8:72–81.
6. Andrade MGS, Weissman R, Oliveira MG, Heitz C. Tooth displacement and root dilacerations after trauma to primary predecessor: an evaluation by computed tomography. Dent Traumatol 2007;23:364–367.
7. Segal GR, Schiffman PH, Tuncay OC. Meta analysis of the treatment-related factors of external apical root resorption. Orthod Craniofacial Res 2004;7:71–78.
8. Jönsson A, Malmgren O, Levander E. Long-term follow-up of tooth mobility in maxillary incisors with orthodontically induced apical root resorption. Eur J Orthod 2007;29:482–487.
9. Kolokitha OE, Papadopoulou AK. Impaction and apical root angulation of the maxillary central incisors due to supernumerary teeth: combined surgical and orthodontic treatment. Am J Orthod Dentofacial Orthop 2008;134:153–160.
10. Kuvvetly SS, Seymen F, Gencay K. Management of an unerupted dilacerated maxillary central incisor: a case report. Dent Traumatol 2007;23:257–261.

11

Premolar Autotransplantation After Avulsion of Both Maxillary Central Incisors

Luc C. Martens

Key words: incisor loss, dental trauma, autotransplantation

Age category: 7–12 years

Definition

Autotransplantation of premolars to replace missing teeth in growing individuals has been shown to be a predictable method with potential for bone induction and re-establishment of a normal alveolar process. From a long-term perspective (20–40 years), transplanted teeth compare favorably with other treatment modalities for substitution of missing teeth when the roots are partly developed. Although autotransplantation has historically been popular in northern European countries, this could be related to the dentists' training background, which was based on a closer relationship between dental surgery and medicine. Nowadays autotransplantation is used worldwide and is a highly suitable treatment for anterior tooth loss.[1]

The recent popularity of implants could probably result in transplantation being overlooked as a further treatment option. However, it should be kept in mind that the optimal time for this treatment is in early childhood, a period where implants are definitely contraindicated.

Key Message

Keeping natural teeth in the alveolar bone instead of movable prosthetic appliances favors the development of the alveolar process. Due to the unique osteogenic capacity of the autograft, this procedure offers a treatment alternative where both the lost tooth and the atrophic alveolar process can be replaced.

THE PROBLEM

A 9-year-old girl presented at the department of oral surgery after a traumatic injury with avulsion of both maxillary central incisors (11, 21). Unfortunately, the avulsed teeth were kept dry and were not cleaned. Both teeth were reimplanted and immobilized with a Schuchardt splint (Fig. 11-1), a method of rigid splinting commonly used by oral surgeons in the late 1970s. Four days after the trauma, both centrals were treated with calcium hydroxide according to the well-known method of M. Cvek. After 6 weeks the splint was removed. Both teeth were neither hypermobile nor sensitive. There were no adverse clinical symptoms. Approximately 1 year after trauma, the patient consulted the orthodontic department for crowding in the mandibular arch.

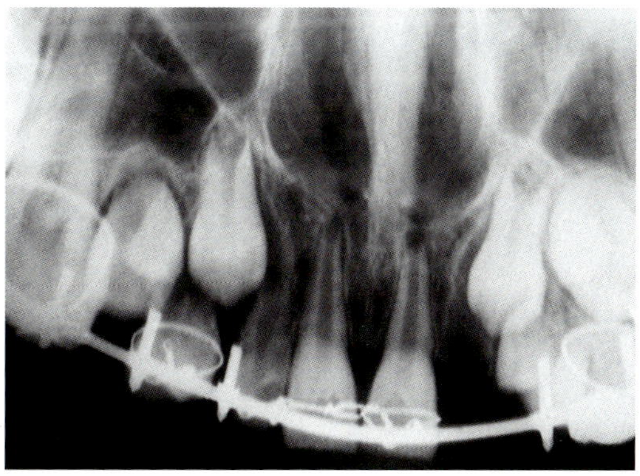

Fig. 11-1 The two reimplanted maxillary central incisors were splinted by means of a Schuchardt splint.

CASE DESCRIPTION

Medical History

ASA I. The child was generally healthy, with no remarkable medical history. There was no history of allergic reactions or medication intake.

Examination

The dentition was complete, except for a missing maxillary lateral incisor, and healthy without any caries lesions and was free of restorations. No visible plaque was present. There was a mild skeletal Class II relationship and a tendency toward vertical growth. There was no overjet or overbite. There was crowding in the mandibular arch, with blocked out canines (33, 43) (Fig. 11-2).

Additional Investigations

The radiographs revealed partial resorption and ankylosis of both the maxillary central incisors (11, 21) (Fig. 11-3).

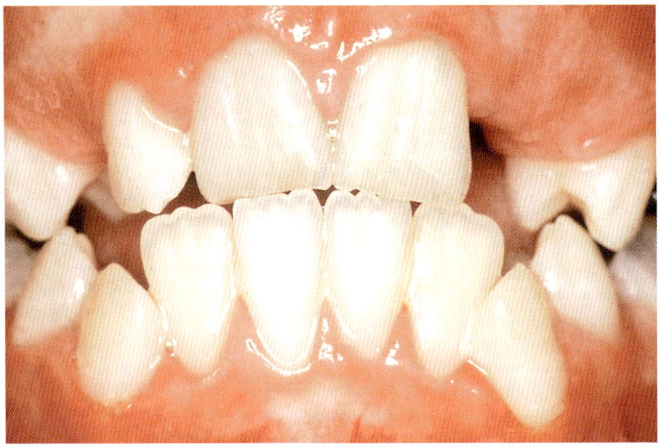

Fig. 11-2 Anterior intraoral view of the reimplanted central incisors (11, 21). Neither overjet nor overbite is present. Note the blocked out mandibular canines (33, 43).

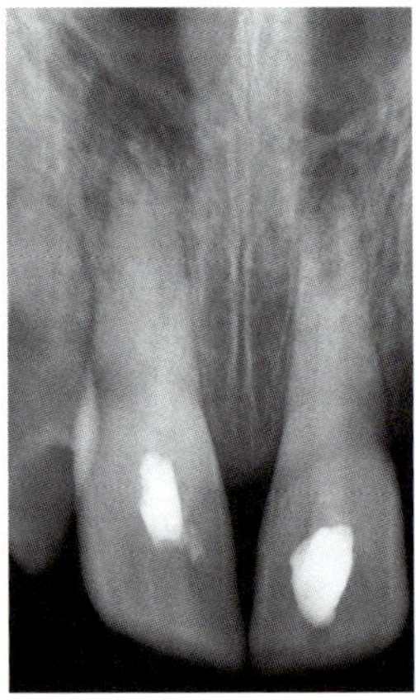

Fig. 11-3 The reimplanted central incisors were endodontically treated. The radiograph shows slight evidence of resorption and ankylosis.

TREATMENT AIM

Taking into account the poor prognosis of both central maxillary incisors, the aim of treatment was premolar transplantation.

TREATMENT OPTIONS

Definitive

While the most frequent indication for premolar transplantation appeared to be agenesis of permanent premolars, a condition which is seen in 6–10% of the population, clearly congenital or accidental loss of anterior teeth is also proving a popular indication. Avulsion of anterior permanent teeth due to trauma occurs in 0.2% of school-age children and a congenital lack of lateral incisors is found in 2% of the general population.[2]

Alternatives

When parents or patients refuse autotransplantation, one should keep in mind that in cases such as the present patient, most probably the central incisors will not survive. At a young age, there is no other solution than prosthetic replacement with removable appliances. In older patients (+18 years), fixed bridgework or implants can be considered.

Rationale

Considering the orthodontic findings, including crowding in the mandibular arch, and the above-mentioned poor prognosis of the maxillary central incisors, it was decided that autotransplantation was the best solution. The age of the patient and the appropriate developmental stage of the premolars were also in favor of this treatment option.

TREATMENT AND FOLLOW-UP

Treatment

At the age of 10 years and 2 months, the mandibular second premolars were transplanted into the maxillary central incisor region. The amount of root development of both premolars was approximately half the length in a fully developed tooth. Both the developing teeth were carefully removed and placed directly in the sockets of the central incisors immediately after their removal at the appropriate height and supported only with silk sutures (Fig. 11-4). Both teeth were rotated over 180 degrees during the transplantation procedure to permit better alignment in the socket and a better esthetic result after build-up. For reasons of symmetry the single maxillary lateral incisor was extracted. As the child had good oral hygiene, good prognosis was expected.

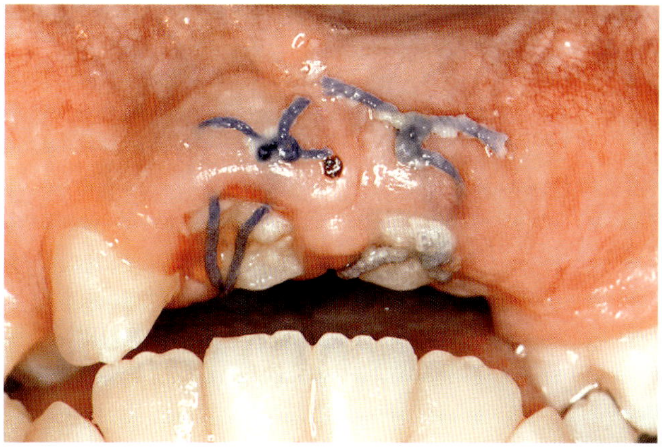

Fig. 11-4 Immediately after transplantation the teeth were supported with silk sutures.

Posttreatment Evaluation/Follow-up

Nine months after transplantation, the clinical crown height of the transplanted premolars was 4 mm and 3.5 mm (Fig. 11-5). Both the transplanted teeth were vital and neither sensitivity nor mobility was noted. The radiographs showed that the pulp canals were still open. Both canines (13, 23) had started to erupt next to the transplanted teeth. Ten months after surgery, the patient presented at the department of pediatric dentistry for the first composite build-up (without any reduction of the transplanted teeth). The esthetic improvement enhanced the child's self-esteem (Fig. 11-6 to Fig. 11-8). Root formation, sensitivity, and mobility were monitored at regular intervals. All outcomes of clinical tests remained normal. Although the premolars showed wide open pulps shortly after transplantation, as the root formation completed, the pulp canals were obliterated (Figs 11-9a, 11-9b). The canines next to the transplanted teeth were moderately reshaped and built with resin composites to resemble the morphologic shape of lateral incisors after full eruption. The final result was an esthetically acceptable maxillary arch with apparently four incisors. In reality no incisor was present.

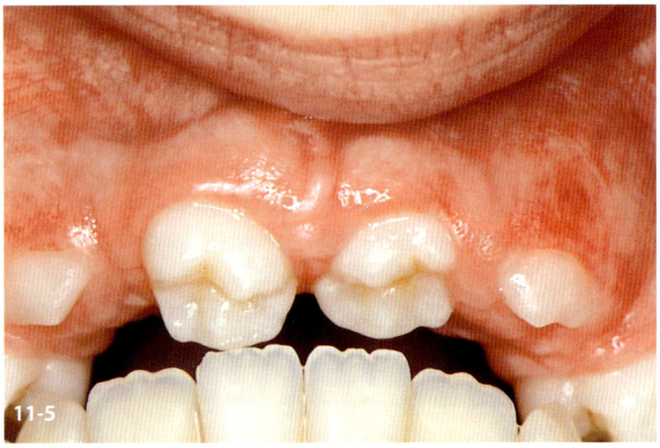

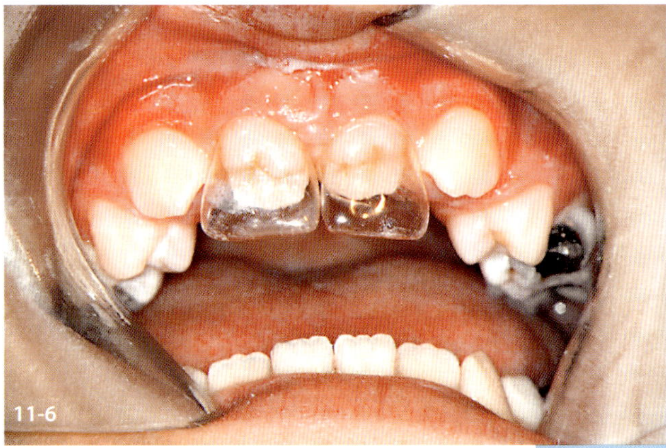

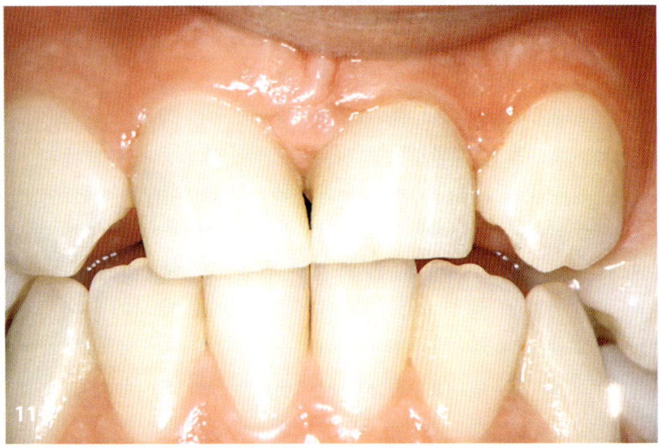

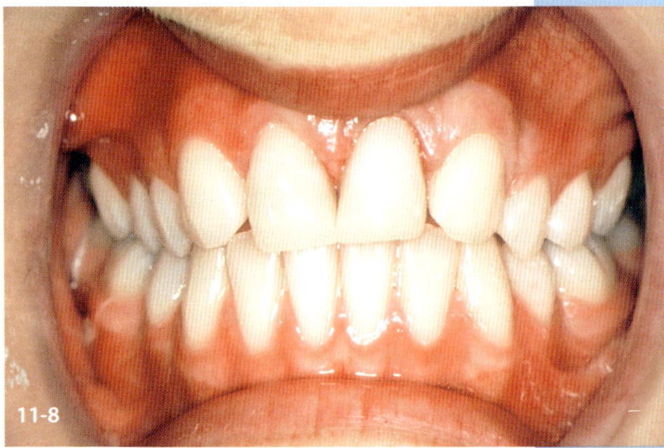

Fig. 11-5 Nine months after transplantation. The canines are erupting next to the transplanted premolars.

Fig. 11-6 Ten months after transplantation. First esthetic build-up using ion crowns.

Fig. 11-7 First stage of esthetic improvement.

Fig. 11-8 Further esthetic improvement after full eruption of the canines.

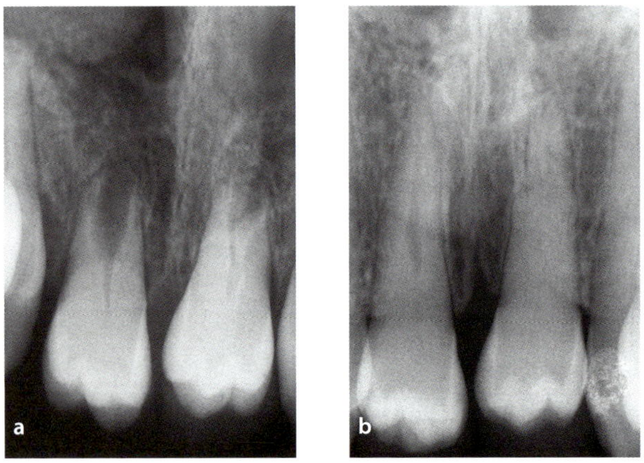

Fig. 11-9a,b The transplanted teeth shortly after surgery. Later radiographs showed completed roots and obliterated pulps.

Crowding in the lower arch resolved spontaneously after removal of both the second premolars (Figs 11-10a, 11-10b). Only two small spaces remained distal to the mandibular first premolars (34, 44) (Figs 11-10c, 11-10d). Three years after transplantation the original plan to use fixed appliances for final alignment was abandoned as further orthodontic treatment did not seem necessary.

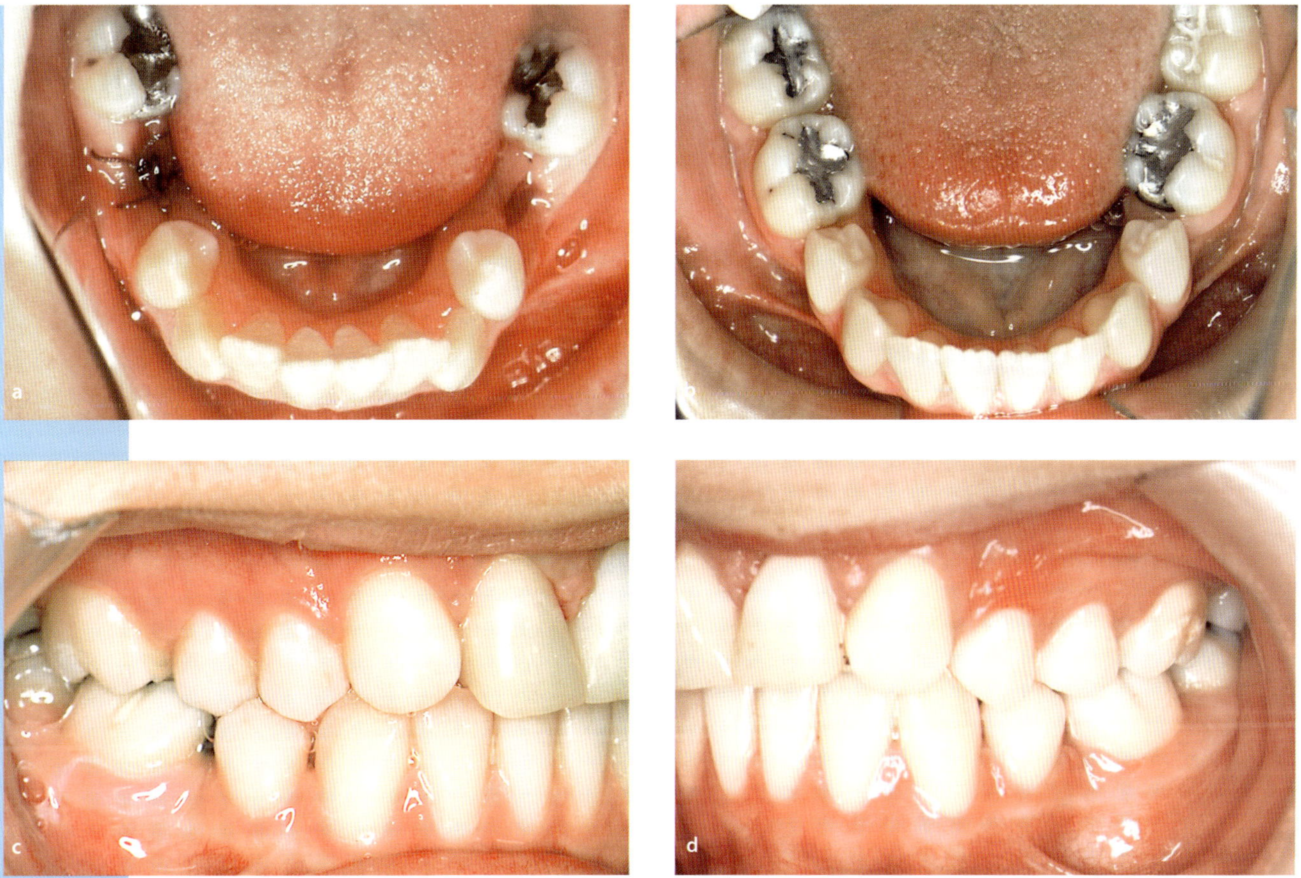

Fig. 11-10a–d Clinical situation immediately after grafting and 2 years after transplantation. A Class I molar relationship has been established. The lower canines aligned spontaneously. Only small interdental spaces remain in the posterior areas.

Both the transplanted premolars remained vital, showed normal physiologic mobility, and were not sensitive after percussion. The buccal segments on both sides showed a Class I molar relationship. The short-term follow-up of this case has been published previously.[3] The patient is now 38 years old, and has had a beautiful smile without any natural incisor for almost 30 years, made possible with her own two transplanted lower second premolars and canines esthetically built up as lateral incisors (Fig. 11-11, Fig. 11-12).

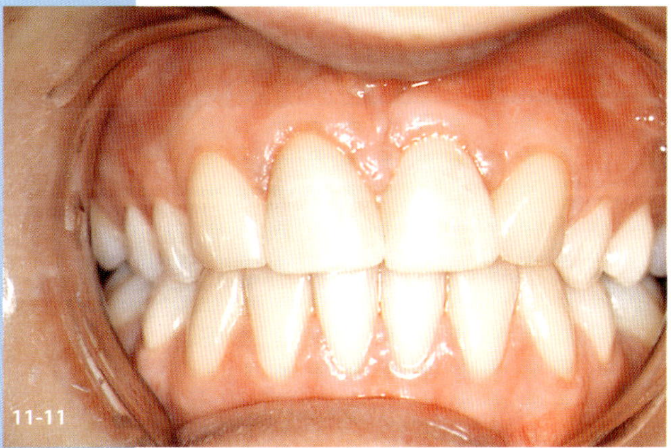

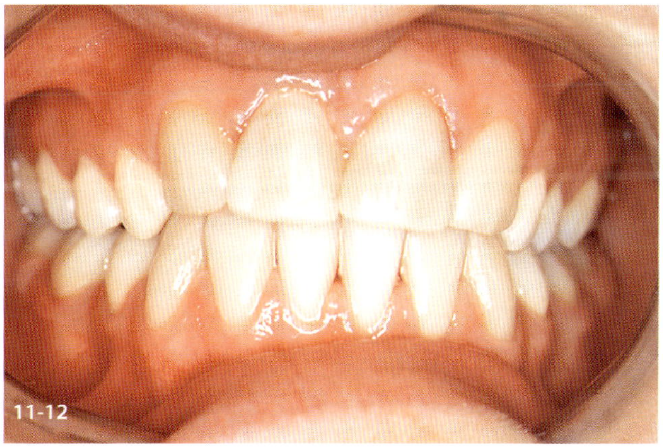

Fig. 11-11 Esthetic improvement, including shaping of the maxillary canines to resemble the lateral incisors.

Fig. 11-12 At 10 years' follow-up.

DISCUSSION

Prognosis after reimplantation depends on a number of factors. The success rate after reimplantation of avulsed teeth, even under ideal circumstances (short extraoral time, no infection, wet conservation), is known to be moderate. The current prognosis data vary enormously with a very large range of:[4]

- tooth survival: 21–89%
- periodontal ligament (PDL) healing: 9–50%
- pulp healing: 4–27%.

In our patient, the conditions were not favorable, which compromised the prognosis. The reimplanted central incisors, however, did maintain the structure of the alveolar process, as well as the space in the central incisor area.

It has been recommended to transplant teeth when the roots have reached one-half to three-quarters of their final length.[1,2] Although in this patient only half of the roots were formed, normal revascularization and an acceptable final root length were expected.

> ***Key Message***
>
> *Besides the developmental stage of the autograft, graft selection is also important.*
>
> *For the replacement of central maxillary incisors, a choice can be made between all premolars except the maxillary first premolars, sometimes the canines, or even small-sized maxillary third molars. For the maxillary lateral incisors only mandibular first premolars should be used. In the canine region, any of the premolars except the maxillary first premolars can be used. It depends on the expertise of the oral surgeon.*

According to Tsukiboshi[5] the following healing processes are the most important predictors of success: PDL healing, bone healing, pulp regeneration, and root development. A number of the factors that are described below can be dealt with by an experienced operator.

Favourable healing of the PDL depends on how many viable cells are preserved on the root. Good PDL healing is expected when a donor tooth is immediately placed into the freshly extracted recipient tooth socket. Besides PDL recovery, the healing of the mechanically damaged root surface with new cementum and PDL is also important. If this does not happen (eg, in the case of inflammation) several processes can occur: root surface resorption, replacement resorption (ankylosis), and finally inflammatory resorption.

Bone healing. The PDL of a transplanted tooth appears to be able to induce bone production. Genetically, PDL cells can differentiate into three types of cell: fibroblasts, cementoblasts, and osteoclasts. The differentiated osteoblast may generate bone around the transplanted tooth.

Pulp regeneration can be expected after replantation and transplantation of teeth with incomplete root formation (ie, a radiographic diameter of the apical foramen of ≥ 1 mm). The invading cells will differentiate into the cells of a functioning pulp. Pulp canal obliteration, however, is inevitable later (as seen in this case).

Root development after transplantation (as seen in this case) can be expected to continue if a donor is immature and Hertwig's epithelial sheath is preserved around the apices. However, the amount of root development to be expected cannot be predicted by the stage of root development of the donor tooth. Ideally, one would wish to transplant a tooth that has reached its maximal length but still has the potential for pulp regeneration (see above). Transplantation of a tooth with a fully formed root eliminates the potential for pulp regeneration, although adequate endodontic therapy will still ensure success. In the present case, the apical foramen was wide open.

Key Message

The strongest predictor for optimal healing of an autotransplanted tooth appears to be the stage of root development and the apical diameter at the time of grafting. A significant factor appears to be the experience of the oral surgeon, and finally, a structured follow-up regimen to monitor periodontal and pulpal conditions seems to be important. The latter has been found to increase the survival rate of autotransplantation to 30%.

Studies worldwide have demonstrated good long-term survival of such transplanted teeth, thus providing a realistic alternative for tooth replacement in young individuals (see Table 11-1). The final prognosis for autotransplantation of teeth in the anterior region is actually estimated to be 98–99% for 5-year and 87–95% for 10-year graft survival.[1]

Table 11-1 Comparison of the cost-effectiveness of different treatment options for anterior tooth loss[1]

	Orthodontics	Implants	Resin-retained bridges	Conventional bridges	Autotransplantation
Cost	+++	+++	+	+++	+
Long-term service	+++	+++	+	++	+++
Use in growing individuals	+++	0	+++	0	+++
Bone-inducing potential	0	0	0	0	+++

0, not be used or non-existent; +, minimum (low); ++, medium (moderate); +++, maximum (high).

Esthetics

Regardless of the method of substitution, the esthetic appearance of single tooth replacements in the incisor area always requires the particular attention of the clinician, since the neighboring, natural teeth are present for immediate comparison. Even if the result is satisfactory from a biologic perspective, the treatment may not be considered successful if the esthetic outcome is less than optimal. So far, no systematic review has been published on the esthetic results and on patients' perceptions when missing teeth are replaced by transplanted premolars. One of the few studies, on 22 transplanted premolars, revealed that for about a quarter of the patients, the esthetic result was unsatisfactory.[6]

Future Perspectives

When a tooth cannot be transplanted immediately, cryopreservation and storage in a tooth bank offers new possibilities for future autotransplantation. An experimental study in dogs showed that teeth can revascularize after transplantation if the original pulp tissue is removed at the time of extraction. Further, there was no significant difference in revascularization between teeth stored in a tooth bank for 7 days and those immediately transplanted without freezing, and there was no difference in the ingrowth of new pulpal tissue between mature apicectomized teeth and immature teeth.[7] Furthermore, a recent literature review concluded that cryopreservation has no negative influence on the repair of the PDL.[8] These results are promising for future clinical considerations in humans.

REFERENCES

1. Andreasen JO, Andersson L, Tsukiboshi M. Autostransplantation of Teeth to the anterior region. In: Andreasen et al. Traumatic Injuries to the Teeth, 4th ed. Oxford: Blackwell-Munksgaard, 2007.
2. Andreasen J. Atlas of Replantation and Transplantation of teeth. Mediglobe SA, 1992.
3. Dermaut L, Verrue V, De pauw G. Transplantation after upper incisor trauma. A case report. Am J Orthod Dentofac Orthop 1994;105:425–429.
4. Andreasen JO, Andreasen FM. Avulsion. In: Andreasen et al. Traumatic Injuries to the Teeth, 4th ed. Oxford: Blackwell-Munksgaard, 2007.
5. Tsukiboshi M. Autotransplantation of teeth: requirements for predictable success. Dent Traumatol 2002;18:157–180.
6. Csochowska EM, Stenvik A, Zachrisson BU. The esthetic outcome of autotransplanted premolars replacing maxillary incisors. Dent Traumatol 2002;18:237–245.
7. Laureys W, Beele H, Cornelissen R, Dermaut L. Revascularization after cryopreservation and autotansplantation of immature and mature apicoectomized teeth. Am J Orthod Dentofac Orthop 2001;119:346–352.
8. Temmerman L, De Pauw G, Beele H, Dermaut L. Tooth transplantation and cryopreservation: state of the art. Am J Orthod Dentofac Orthop 2006;129:691–695.

12

Prosthetic Rehabilitation in a Patient With Ectodermal Dysplasia

Andrea Savi
Manfredi Maddalena
Marco Tamani
Mario Fazzi
Silvia Pizzi

Key words: ectodermal dysplasia, prosthetic rehabilitation, denture

Age category: 4–7 years

Definition

Ectodermal dysplasia (ED) is a hereditary disease characterized by congenital dysplasia of two or more ectodermal structures, such as skin, hair, nails, and eccrine sweat glands. In addition, other defects in the external morphology (nose, outer ears, lips), in the central nervous system (CNS), alterations of the eyes, and anomalies in the oronasal mucosa and melanocytes have been described. The most frequently observed form of ED is X-linked hypohidrotic (anhidrotic) ED (Christ–Siemens–Touraine syndrome), first described in 1848 and characterized by the triad of hypotrichosis (skin, hair, and nail anomalies), either hypodontia or anodontia, hypohidrosis (partial or total absence of eccrine sweat glands), and other features such as prominent supraorbital ridges, frontal bossing, and a saddle-shaped nose. A second type of ED, named hidrotic ED, has also been described.[1–6]

Numerous combinations of the clinical manifestations may present in ED, with up to 154 different types and 11 subgroups, labeled from 1 to 4 according to whether they affect the hair, teeth, nails, or sweat glands. The diagnosis of patients with ED is mainly based on the clinical history, skin biopsy in cases of changes in sweating, hair study, and molecular genetic analysis.[4,6]

THE PROBLEM

Ronnie (age 6) was referred by his geneticist to the dentistry unit at the University of Parma for dental evaluation and prosthetic rehabilitation owing to the non-eruption of his permanent teeth. The patient had a subtype of ED. At this time, he was starting to become uncomfortable with the appearance of his teeth and was very reluctant to smile. He was very motivated to undergo dental rehabilitation.

CASE DESCRIPTION

History

Medical History

Ronnie was diagnosed as having ED with an autosomal-dominant mode of inheritance, incomplete penetrance (which occurs when some individuals fail to express the trait even though they carry the allele), and variable expressivity (which occurs when a phenotype is expressed to a different degree among individuals with the same genotype). (Apart from severe hypodontia [only two teeth were present], frontal bossing and everted lips in profile, his phenotype was not typical of ED; in particular no nail, skin, or hair anomalies were recorded. Ronnie also had mild mental retardation and hypoacusia (hearing impediment). According to the family history, other members of his mother's family were affected by hypodontia (grandmother and aunts); however, a family tree/inheritance schedule was not available at the time of the dental examinations. His mother had hip dysplasia, dry skin, and a mental disorder.

Dental History
Dental records revealed a severe case of hypodontia: only two mandibular primary teeth were present. The patient resembled an elderly edentulous person (Figs 12-1a, 12-1b).

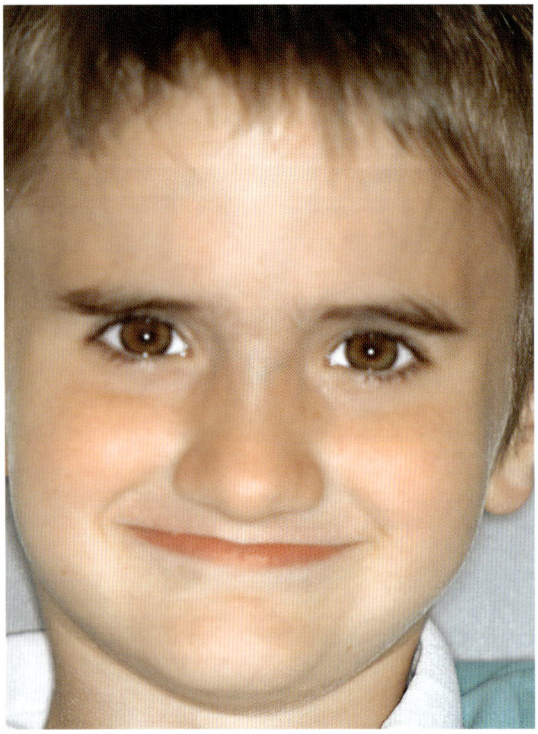

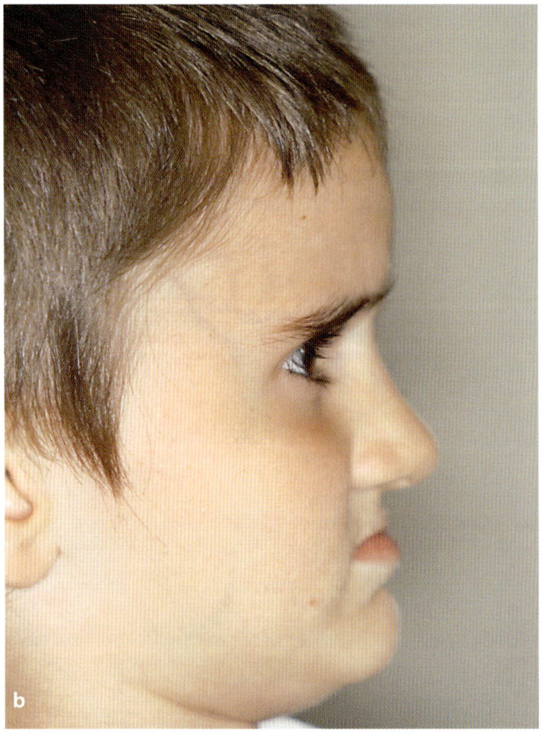

Fig. 12-1a,b Anterior and profile views of the patient.

Oral Hygiene
Ronnie's oral hygiene was good at the time of the first clinical examination. He and his family were very keen on prosthetic treatment and this had a good influence on oral hygiene practices. However, periodic checkups were prescribed in order to monitor oral health status as well as to make small adjustments and modifications to the prosthesis, especially the mandibular denture.

Examination
On intraoral examination, there were only two permanent teeth in the mandible; all the other teeth were missing. The appearance of the alveolar and gingival mucosa was normal although the alveolar ridges were atrophic, except for the posterior mandibular areas, where the two first permanent molars (36, 46) were present. The vertical dimension of occlusion was reduced, as evidenced by deep folds in the commissures of the mouth and the thin lips (Fig. 12-2, Fig. 12-3).

Additional Investigations
A panoramic radiograph confirmed that the patient had only two permanent teeth (the two mandibular first molars) in the mandible. In the maxilla all of the anterior and posterior permanent tooth germs were missing (Fig. 12-4).

> ***Key Message***
> *ED is an inherited syndrome in which two or more ectodermal structures fail to develop. Hypodontia is observed in patients with dental anomalies.*

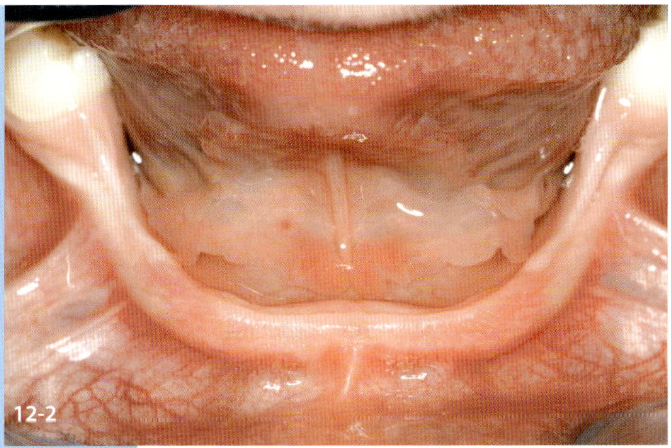

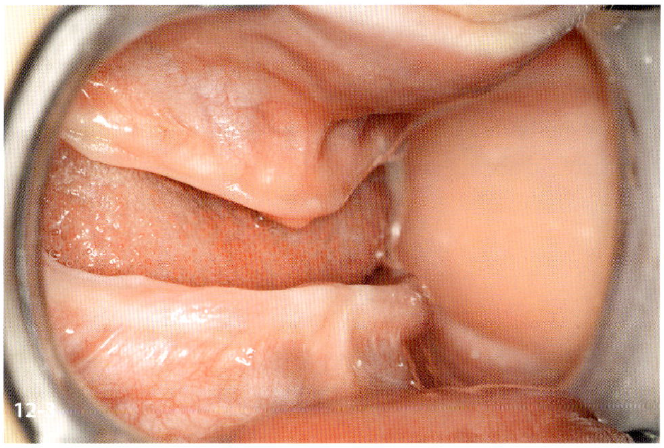

Fig. 12-2 Intraoral view of the edentulous mandibular alveolar crest.

Fig. 12-3 Vertical jaw inter-relationship.

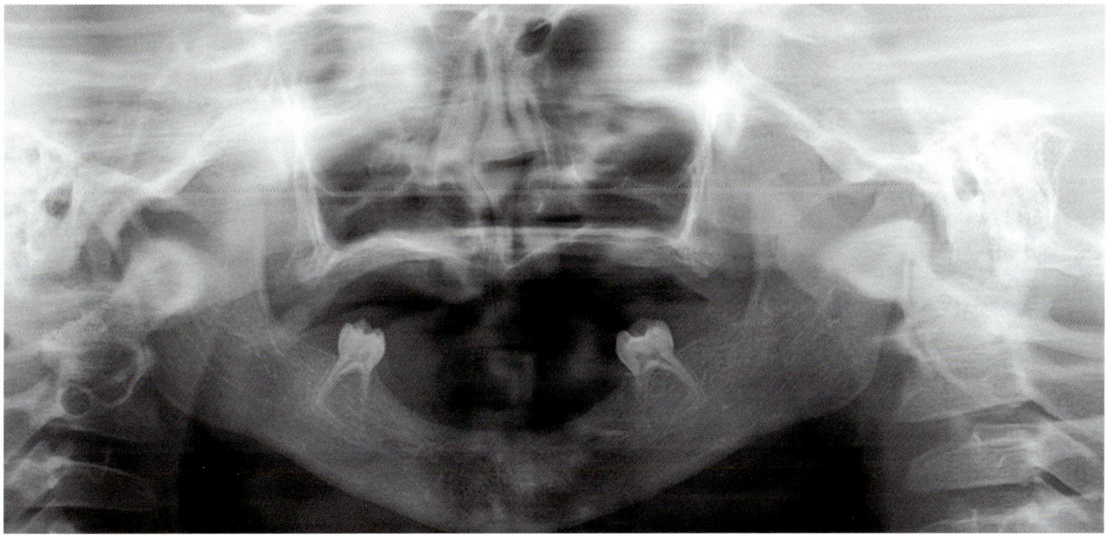

Fig. 12-4 Panoramic radiograph showing the presence of only two teeth (two permanent molars).

TREATMENT AIM

The aim of the treatment was oral rehabilitation, using two removable dentures.

TREATMENT OPTIONS

Definitive

- Full mouth prosthetic rehabilitation with a complete maxillary dental prosthesis and a partial mandibular denture.

New dental prostheses were planned to maintain the appearance of mixed dentition compatible with a child of Ronnie's age. In addition, mini-implants were planned to better stabilize the prostheses, as a provisional step in preparation for the definitive implant treatment when the jaws had fully developed.

Alternatives

- Full mouth rehabilitation with endosseous dental implants.

Rationale

Conventional prosthodontic treatment for patients with ED has consisted of various combinations of overdentures, complete or partial removable prostheses, and fixed prostheses. Recently, endosseous dental implants have been reported to be a good alternative for patients affected by this condition, to support and stabilize the dental prosthesis. These treatment strategies can be used individually or in combination to achieve an optimal result. However, because of the early age at the time of initial intervention and the need to easily modify the prosthesis during the child's growth period, a removable (partial/complete) denture is initially preferable.[1]

TREATMENT AND FOLLOW-UP

Treatment

A complete maxillary removable denture and partial mandibular denture were made for the patient. At the time of treatment planning, cephalometric analysis, which involves the assessment of the relationship of the jaws, was performed to help minimize potential interferences as the child grew. In particular, two- and three-way orthodontic expanders were placed within the mandibular and maxillary removable prostheses to ensure denture expansion to accommodate subsequent skeletal growth. The dentures greatly improved the patient's appearance and jaw function. Periodic follow-ups were prescribed, initially every week, then once a month and then every 6 months, to monitor oral hygiene and to make adjustments and modifications to the prosthesis (Fig. 12-5 to Fig. 12-10).

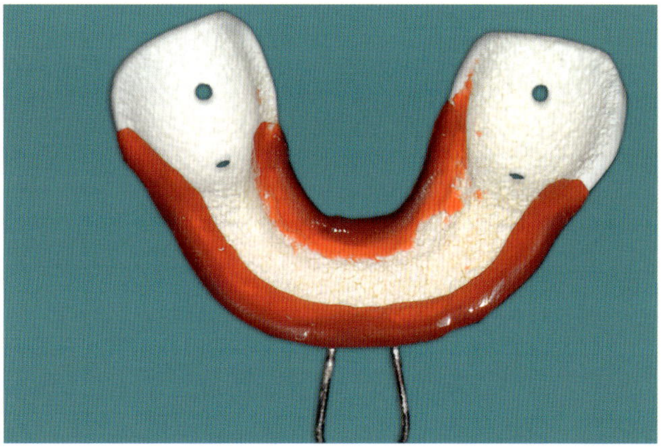

Fig. 12-5 Individual tray.

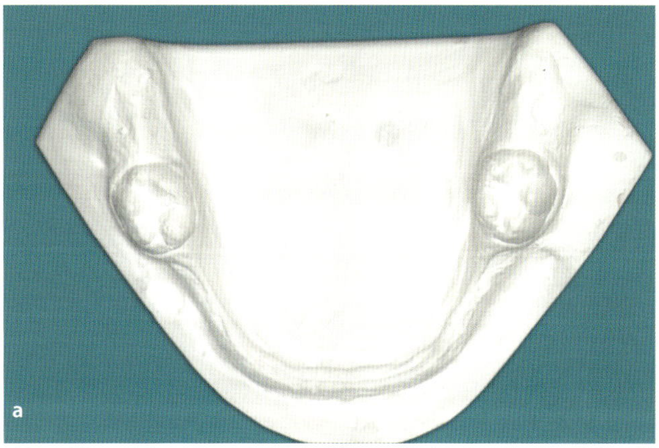

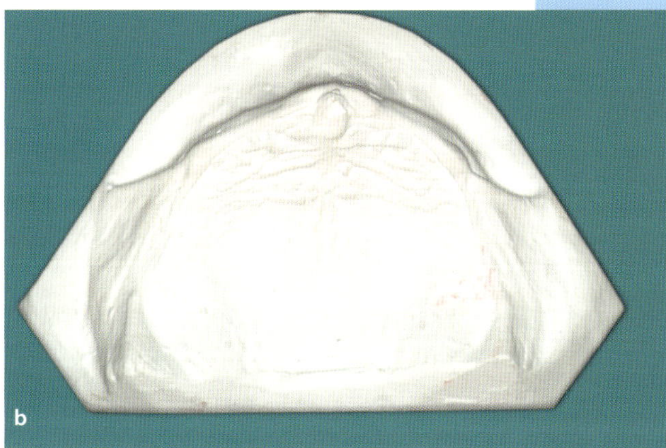

Fig. 12-6a,b Mandibular and maxillary casts.

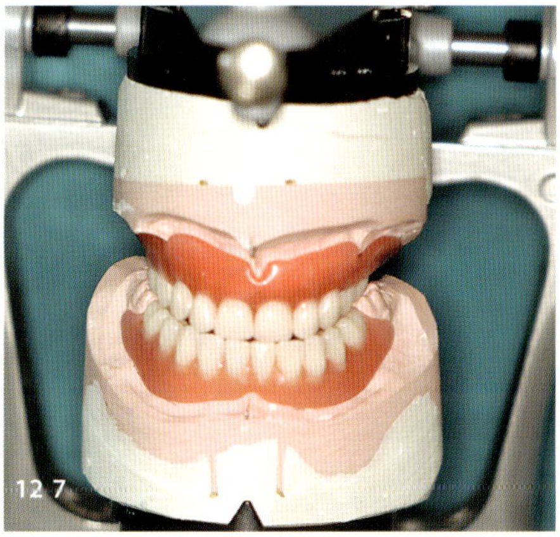

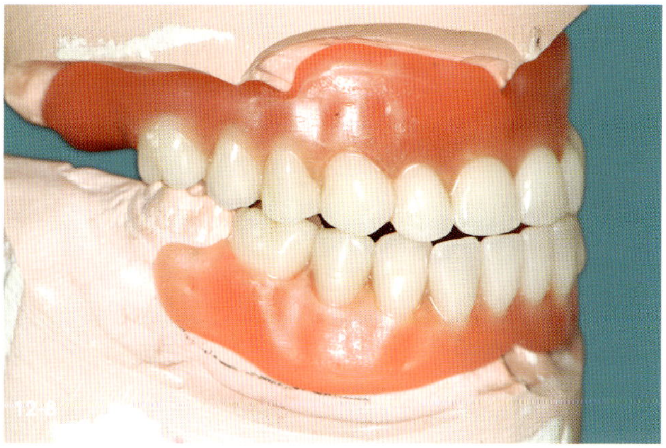

Fig. 12-7 Dental casts mounted on an articulator.

Fig. 12-8 Occlusal relationships of the dentures.

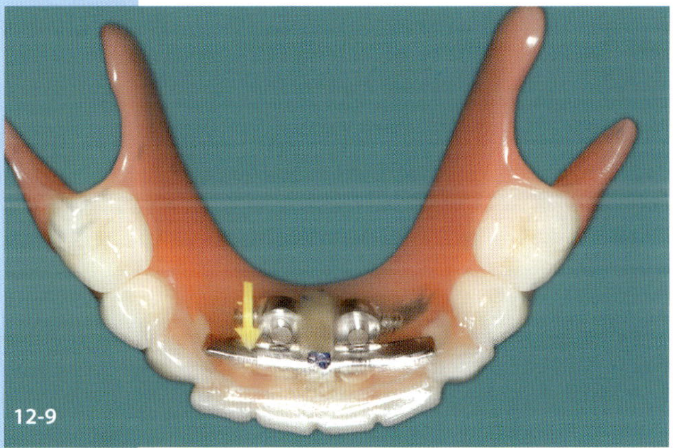

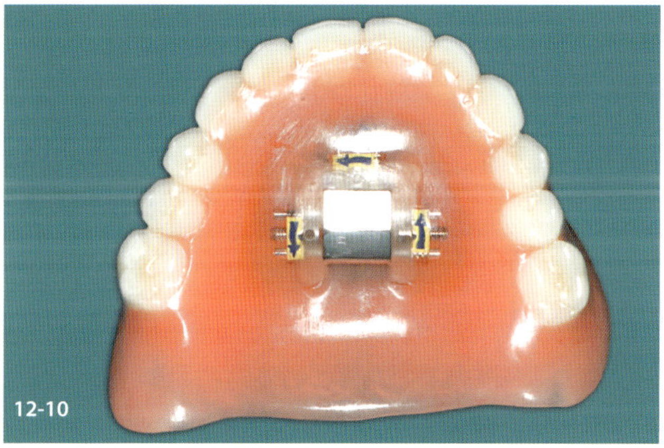

Fig. 12-9 Mandibular partial denture.

Fig. 12-10 Maxillary complete denture.

Posttreatment Evaluation/Follow-up

One year later, the patient had adapted well to his dentures and the treatment had improved his masticatory and speech function, and appearance. His self-esteem (assessed by discussion with parents and school teachers) had also improved and he seemed happy to smile (Fig. 12-11, Fig. 12-12).

DISCUSSION

ED is characterized by severe congenital and developmental anomalies. Hypodontia/anodontia is the most common oral feature of this condition. These anomalies affect esthetics and function, which can further affect the psychosocial status of these patients.[1] Therefore, when treating a child with ED, it is important to motivate both the patient as well as their family in order to evaluate their compliance. Treatment of ED may include the use of removable and/or fixed partial dentures, complete denture prosthesis, or implant-retained prosthesis when possible. Each treatment approach can be used individually or in combination to obtain an optimal result. Owing to the young age of these patients, atrophy of alveolar bone and on-going development of the jaws, the use of removable prostheses is recommended during the first stages of treatment (3–6 years).[6] The use of endosseous dental implants should be delayed until a more stable vertical dimension and jaw interrelationship are established,[1,8] which normally occurs at 18 years of age. Prosthetic rehabilitation

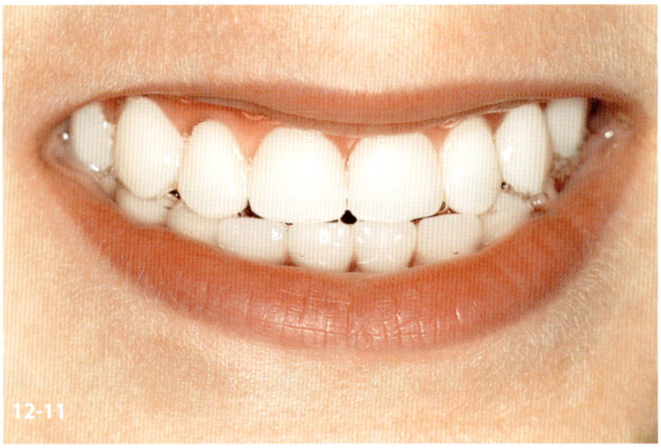

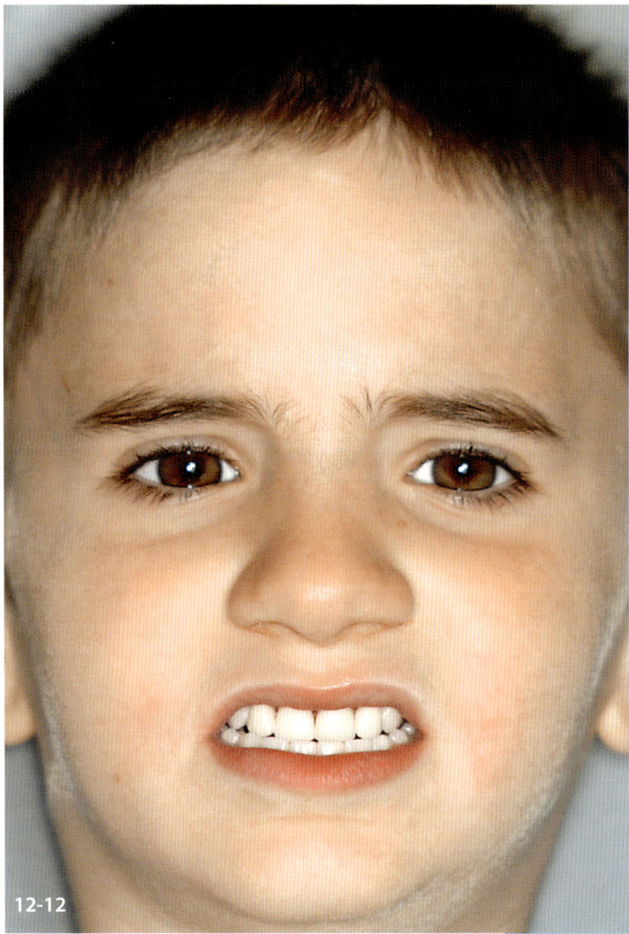

Fig. 12-11 Intraoral view of the prostheses.

Fig. 12-12 Patient with the two prostheses in situ.

should be initiated as soon as possible to avoid possible bone resorption and to control the vertical dimension, which is affected by the lack of teeth.

Oral discomfort may be reported by anhidrotic patients who are using prosthetic appliances, as well as the development of *Candida* spp. superinfection (eg, denture stomatitis associated with *Candida* spp.) In order to avoid these situations, careful oral and prosthetic hygiene is recommended, as well as the use of saliva substitutes.

REFERENCES

1. Bal C, Bal BT, Tufekçiogiu D. Treatment consideration for a patient with hypohidrotic ectodermal dysplasia: a case report. J Contemp Dent Pract 2008;9:1–7.
2. Campuzano S, Santos-Juanes J, Medina A, Sanchez J. Dysplasia ectodermica hipohidrotica. Ann Pediatr 2005;62:393–394.
3. Della Valle D, Chevitarese AB, Maia LC, Farinhas JA. Alternative rehabilitation treatment for a patient with ectodermal dysplasia. J Clin Pediatr Dent 2004;28:103–106.
4. Pinheiro M, Freire-Maia N. Ectodermal dysplasias: a clinical classification and a causal review. Am J Med Genet 1994;53:153–162.
5. Rad AS, Siadat H, Monzavi A, Mangoli A. Full mouth rehabilitation of a hypohidrotic ectodermal dysplasia patient with dental implants: a clinical report. J Prosthodont 2007;16:209–213.
6. Vallejo PA, Lopez-Arranz Monje E, Gonzalez Garcia M, Miguel Martinez F, Blanco-Moreno Alvarez Buylla F. Treatment with removable prosthesis in hypohidrotic ectodermal dysplasia. A clinical case. Med Oral Patol Oral Cir Bucal 2008;13:E119–123.
7. Pavarina AC, Machado AL, Vergani CE, Giampaolo ET. Overlay partial denture for a patient with ectodermal dysplasia: a clinical report. J Prosthet Dent 2001;86:574–577.
8. Sweeney IP, Ferguson JW, Heggie AA, Lucas JO. Treatment outcomes for adolescent ectodermal dysplasia patients treated with dental implants. Int J Clin Pediatr Dent 2005;15:241–248.

13

Tongue Piercing

Roeland De Moor

Key words: abrasion, mucogingival defect, speech interference, oral complications, tongue piercing, tooth fracture

Age category: 12–18 years

Definition

Body piercing is defined as "a penetration of jewelry into openings made in such body areas as eyebrows, helix of the ears, lips, tongue, nose, navel, nipples, and genitals" and is a cultural practice that dates back to antiquity. Body piercing and other body modifications have increased tremendously in popularity in recent years, and have started to be practiced across many social and age groups. Of significance for the dental profession is the increasing popularity of tongue and lip piercings, which is the insertion of jewelry into the oral soft tissues, including the lips, cheeks, and tongue. Rarely it may also involve other sites such as the uvula. It appears that the tongue is the most prevalent oral piercing site, typically pierced in the midline and just anterior to the lingual frenum. Most oral jewelry comes in the form of studs, hoops or barbell-shaped devices that can be purchased commercially. Surgical-grade stainless steel, 14-karat yellow or white gold or niobium oral jewelry is recommended.[1]

The first report of oral body piercing was published in 1992,[2] but it was not until 1997 that the seriousness of potential complications became apparent when spreading infection compromised a patient's airway.[3] Later publications listed around 18 complications, which ranged from the minor inconvenience of the obstruction of radiographic images to the potentially life-threatening, such as prolonged bleeding.[4–7] The death of a Sheffield teenager following lip piercing was debated in the UK Parliament in February 2003.[8] Currently, there is an ongoing debate in different countries about whether the insertion of jewelry in the tongue should be prohibited under the age of 18. A number of procedure-related risks have been described: infection, prolonged bleeding, bloodborne disease transmission, endocarditis, injury to gums, damage to teeth (Figs 13-1a to 13-1c, Fig. 13-2), and interference with normal oral function (Figs 13-3a–c), oral health evaluation (Figs 13-4a to 13-4c), and aspiration.[9]

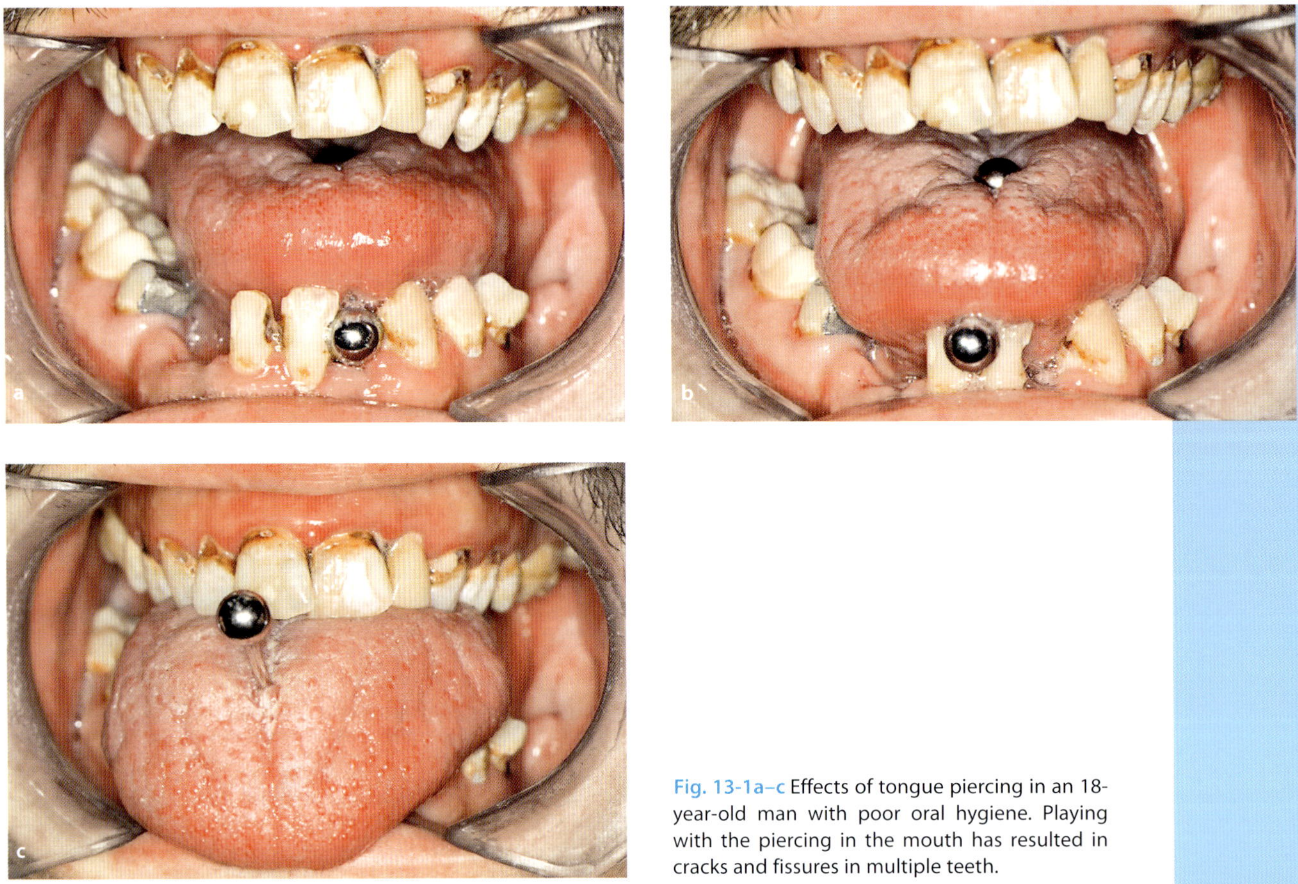

Fig. 13-1a–c Effects of tongue piercing in an 18-year-old man with poor oral hygiene. Playing with the piercing in the mouth has resulted in cracks and fissures in multiple teeth.

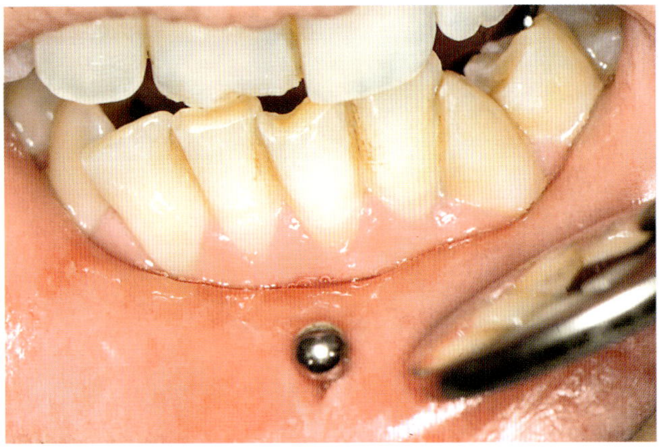

Fig. 13-2 Abrasion lesion on the incisal ridge of the mandibular left central incisor (31) and cracks in the mesioincisal ridge of the maxillary right central incisor (11) due to interposition of the barbell of a lip piercing.

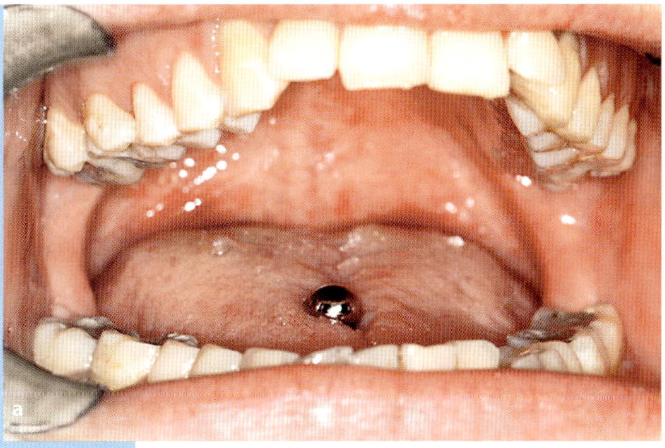

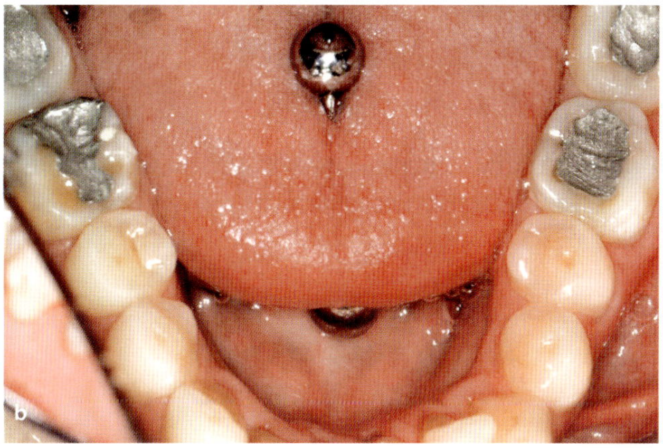

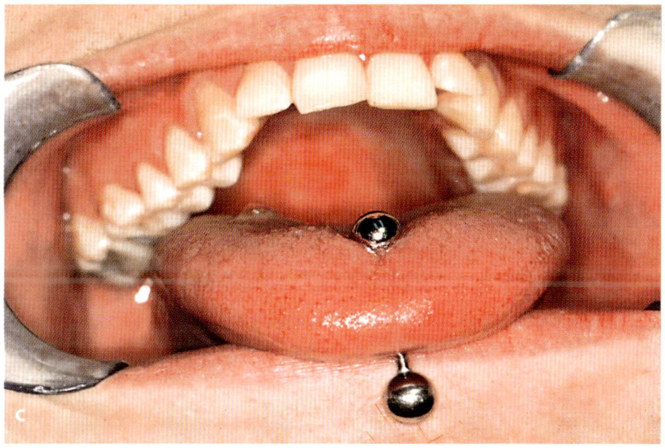

Figs 13-3a–c An 18-year-old patient with speech impediment due to a loose tongue piercing. It was possible to move the piercing all along the oral cavity because of the very long barbell.

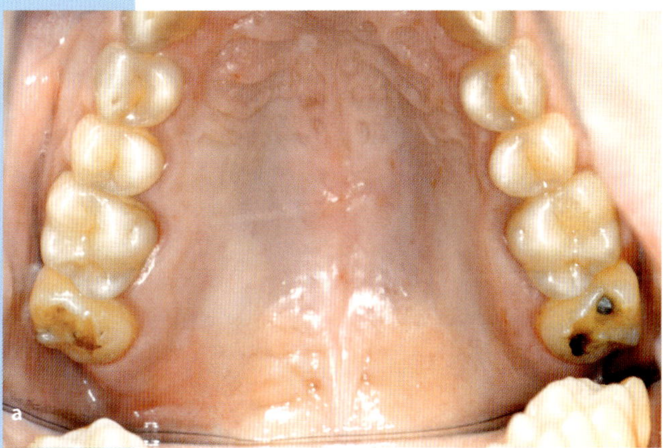

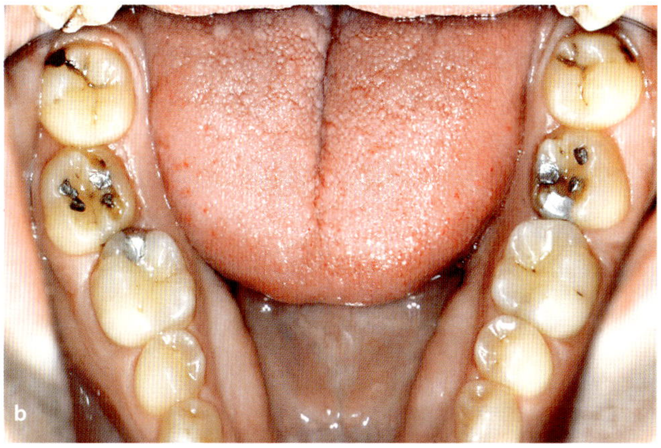

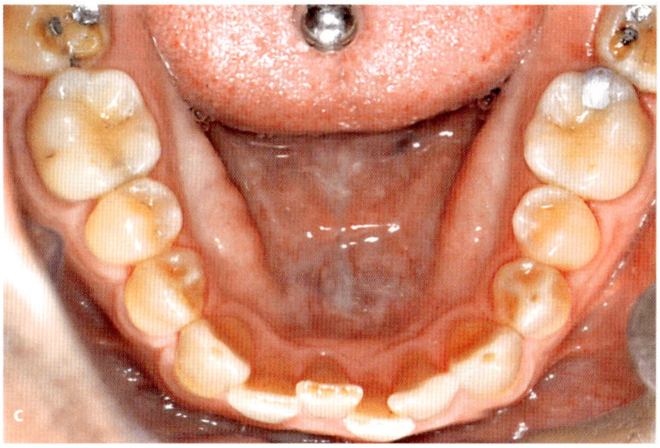

Figs 13-4a–c A diagnostic challenge: 13-4a, 13-4b show the maxillary second molars and the mandibular first molars without occlusal enamel, apparently without any explanation, during a routine checkup. Only after detailed history taking did it became clear that the patient had a tongue piercing, which he had removed for this occasion. With the piercing in place it was clear that the localized abrasions on the surfaces of the molars were the result of abrasion caused by the tongue piercing.

CASE 1

THE PROBLEM

During a routine checkup it was seen that the tongue piercing in 18-year-old Sarah's mouth was associated with scar tissue formation after healing of a prior tear (Fig. 13-5). The piercing had now been in the mouth for 18 months.

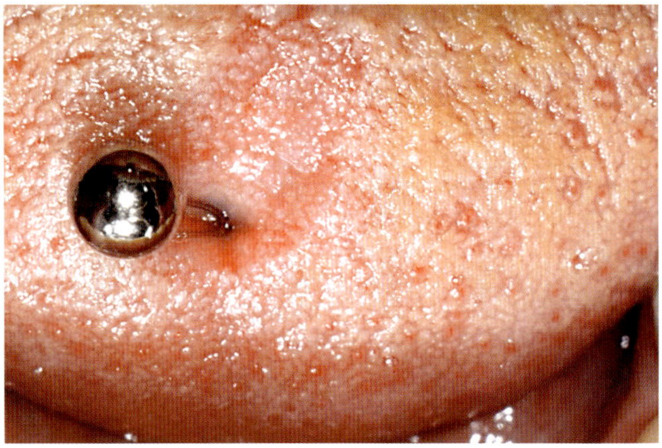

Fig. 13-5 Tear in the tongue with formation of hyperplastic tissue (scar) next to the hole in the tongue.

CASE DESCRIPTION

History

Medical History
ASA I. Sarah was a healthy young woman with no medical problems.

Dental History
Sarah regularly visited her dentist for a checkup. She had good oral hygiene and removed the piercing once a week to be cleaned and disinfected. There was history of persisting swelling and problems with healing after piercing of the tongue. The patient, however, did not consult any medical doctor or dentist, as she was reluctant to confront her parents with these problems as they disapproved of piercing.

Examination
There was hyperplastic tissue around the perforation in the tongue. There were no particular dental problems.

Additional Investigations
Radiographs were taken but did not reveal any signs of pathology or radiolucency that could be associated with cracked teeth or comparable problems. The periodontal condition was good.

TREATMENT AIM

- Convincing the patient to remove the tongue piercing.

TREATMENT OPTIONS

Definitive
Removal of the piercing and the hyperplastic tissue.

Alternatives

If the patient was reluctant to have the piercing removed, it would be more difficult to close the tongue perforation and it would certainly need surgical debridement. In the present case, the piercing was also too loose so that other problems were to be expected: chipping of teeth with eventual fracture, gingival recession because of continuous contact of the piercing with the gingival margins on the lingual aspect of the teeth. Problems with mastication and speech impediments could also follow (especially in pronouncing s, sh, th, ph, t, and v). Speech interference is generally a short-term complication (2–4 weeks) as a result of swelling of the tongue after insertion of the piercing and is found in 14–51% of patients.[5,10] In the present case, the loose tongue piercing should have been replaced by one with a shorter barbell.

Rationale

Oral piercings, although socially acceptable, seem to have serious implications for oral heath status. As the wearing of piercings in the oral cavity can be seen as self-mutilation, maximum effort should be made to prevent oral damage, including taking all oral preventive measures if the piercings are not removed.

The patient was advised that it would be better to remove the hyperplastic tissue and the piercings. However, all attempts at persuasion failed.

PROGNOSIS/FOLLOW-UP

Removal of both the hyperplastic tissue and the piercing should result in spontaneous closure of the tongue perforation in a short period of time.

In the present case it was decided to try to stabilize the situation as the patient refused to have the piercing removed. However, she did not show up for the next checkup.

DISCUSSION

The present patient had good oral health. When hyperplasia is present there is a risk for evolution into a granuloma next to or around the hole. This granuloma, also called pyogenic granuloma, is a common reactive neoformation in the oral cavity that develops in response to local irritation or trauma and is composed of granulation tissue. Various names have been given to this entity, reflecting, in part, mistaken concepts about its etiology and pathogenesis: botryomycosis hominis, botryomycoma, telangiectatic granuloma, benign pedunculated granuloma, fibroangioma, septic granuloma, hemangiomatous granuloma, lobular capillary hemangioma, etc.[11]

The most widely used term is pyogenic granuloma, although it does not adequately describe the lesion's characteristics. The term "pyogenic" implies pus production related to an infectious etiology; however, no pus-producing microorganisms are associated with pyogenic granuloma. Moreover, the lesion is not a true "granuloma" (ie, a specific type of persistent chronic inflammation).

Pyogenic granuloma is not an infectious lesion but a reactive lesion, due to local irritating factors (in this case, tongue piercing). Therefore, it is included in the large group of inflammatory hyperplasias, neoformations due to increase in the number of constituent cells and not genuine tumors in the sense that their excessive growth is not autonomous but depends on a continuous stimulus of traumatic nature.

CASE 2

THE PROBLEM

William (age 18) had hypersensitive teeth with extensive attrition of the incisal edges and occlusal surfaces of the teeth. Moreover, he had localized gingival recession on the buccal aspect of the mandibular left central incisor (31) and limited recession on the buccal aspect of the maxillary left canine (23) (Figs 13-6a to 13-6c).

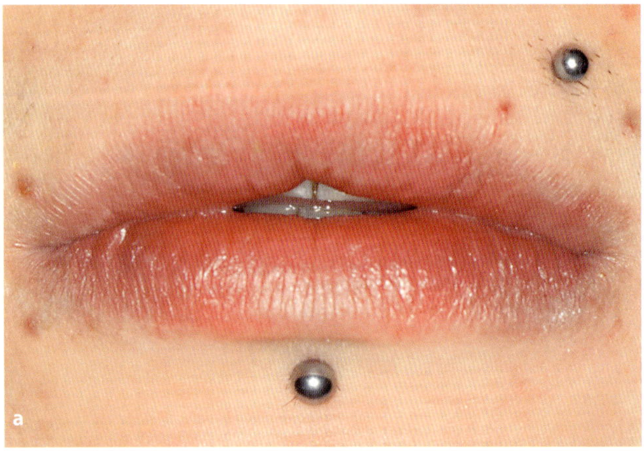

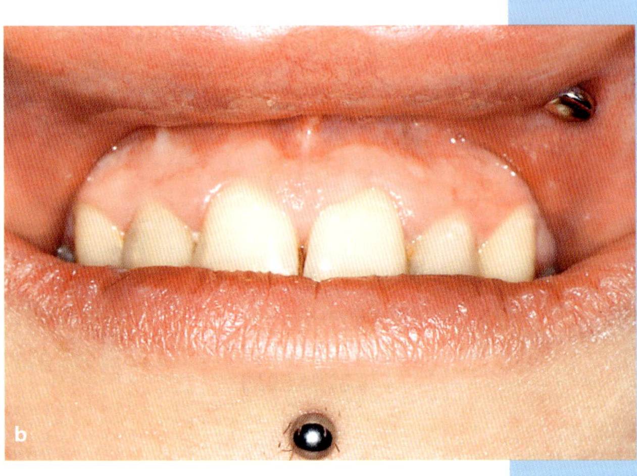

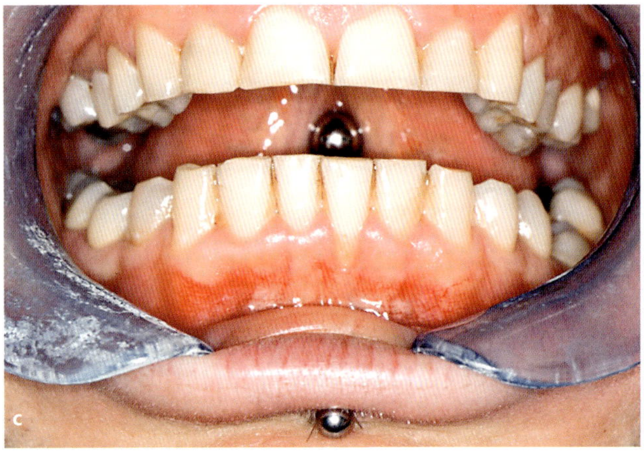

Figs 13-6a–c Extensive incisal and occlusal wear, and localized gingival recession on the buccal aspect of the maxillary left canine (23) and mandibular left central incisor (31). An impression of the stud of the lip piercing in the cervical gingival margin is seen resulting in the start of recession. The recession on the buccal side of the mandibular left central incisor is pronounced and there is clear loss of attachment, exposing the root surface.

CASE DESCRIPTION

History

Medical History
ASA I. William was a healthy young man with strong musculature. He was a keen weight lifter. There were no medical problems.

Dental History
William complained of permanently hypersensitive teeth. He had good oral hygiene but regularly consumed sport drinks.

Examination

There was generalized wear of the incisal edges and occlusal surfaces, although without excessive exposure of dentin. The patient had two lip piercings and one tongue piercing since 1 year. Both lip piercings had resulted in mucogingival damage with exposure of the root of the mandibular left central incisor and early recession with an imprint of the oral part of the lip piercing in the region of the gingival cervical area of the maxillary left canine (23).

TREATMENT AIM

The aim was to protect the teeth from further wear and erosion and reduce the hypersensitivity. The use of sport drinks, which had resulted in erosion, had to be monitored. Removal of the lip piercings was advocated. The tongue piercing has not resulted in any form of oral damage, but William was advised to remove this piercing too (he already removed the tongue piercing during exercise, and reinserted the ornament afterwards). Lussi and colleagues[12] demonstrated that the interplay between erosion and abrasion (in William – acidic beverages together with foreign objects enhancing abrasion) might be the main driver leading to the clinical manifestation of this disorder.

TREATMENT OPTIONS

Definitive

- Removal of the piercings
- Tooth protection by wearing an individualized plastic tray while weight lifting
- Careful use of sport drinks.

Alternative

There were no alternative treatment options.

Rationale

See Case 1, Rationale.

TREATMENT AND FOLLOW-UP

Treatment

The patient was convinced to follow the proposed preventive measures, along with reduction in the hypersensitivity of the teeth, stabilization of the gingival recession after removal of the piercing and the need for coverage of the buccal side of the root of the mandibular left central incisor (31).

Posttreatment Evaluation/Follow-up

The situation was stabilized. For the extensive gingival recession (tooth 31), root coverage (periodontal plastic surgery) will be considered (at present the patient is not in favor of this procedure – "time will tell").

DISCUSSION

Several cases of piercing-associated gingival recession and attachment loss have been documented (on average around 12.5–15% of people with oral piercing claim that they have injuries associated with lip piercing, and 10–20% claim that they have injuries associated with tongue jewelry).[7,13] A cause-and-effect relationship has been found between the barbell's length for the tongue piercing and the size and location of the stud of a lip piercing, and the duration for which the unit was in the mouth and the amount of recession.

REFERENCES

1. Armstrong ML, Ekmark E, Brooks B. Body piercing: promoting informed decision making. J Sch Nurs 1995;11:20–25.
2. Chen M, Scully C. Tongue piercing – a new fad in body art. Br Dent J 1992;172:87.
3. Perkins CS, Meisner J, Harrison JM. A complication of tongue piercing. Br Dent J 1997;182:147–148.
4. De Moor RJG, De Witte AMJC, De Bruyne MAA. Tongue piercing and associated oral and dental complications. Endod Dent Traumatol 2000;16:232–237.
5. De Moor RJG, De Witte AMJC, Delmè KIM, De Bruyne MAA, Hommez GMG, Goyvaerts D. Dental and oral complications of lip and tongue piercings. Br Dent J 2005;199:506–509.
6. Stirn A. Body piercing: medical consequences and psychological motivations. Lancet 2003;361:1205–1215.
7. Levin L, Zadik Y. Oral piercing: complications and side effects. Am J Dent 2007;20:340–344.
8. United Kingdom Parliament. Body piercing. Hansard (House of Commons Daily Debates) 2003;400:27. Available from: www.publications.parliament.uk (accessed 11 September 2008).
9. ADA Division of Communications. Oral piercing and health. J Am Dent Assoc 2001;132:127.
10. Stead LR, Williams JV, Williams AC, Robinson CM. An investigation into the practice of tongue piercing in the South West of England. Br Dent J 2006;200:103–107.
11. Jafarzadeh H, Santkhani M, Mohtasham N. Oral pyogenic granuloma: a review. J Oral Sci 2006;48:167–175.
12. Lussi A, Jaeggi T, Zero D. The role of diet in the aetiology of dental erosion. Caries Res 2004;38(suppl. 1):34–44.
13. Brooks JK, Hooper K, Reynolds MA. Formation of mucogingival defects associated with intraoral and perioral piercing. J Am Dent Assoc 2003;134:837–843.

14

Complicated Crown Fractures in Two Permanent Incisors

Ilija Skrinjaric

Key words: complicated crown fractures, permanent incisors, pulp capping, partial pulpotomy, Cvek pulpotomy

Definition

Complicated crown fractures involve enamel–dentin and pulp. At the site of a pulp exposure it is possible to observe red pulp tissue or slight hemorrhage from the pulp (see Fig. 14-1d below). If treatment of such injury is delayed for several days in young permanent teeth, proliferation of pulp tissue can occur (ie, pulp polyp). The exposed pulp commonly causes symptoms such as sensitivity to thermal stimuli.[1]

THE PROBLEM

ASA I. Simon (12 years) was referred to the department of pediatric dentistry at the University of Zagreb for injured maxillary permanent incisors. He had thermal sensitivity in the maxillary left central and lateral incisors and a contusion in the chin region. He was under orthodontic treatment for maxillary protrusion (distorelation). His maxillary teeth were bonded with brackets and there was an archwire present.

During break at school he had slipped while playing. He had struck his chin against the floor and sustained soft tissue injury in the chin region and vertical crown fractures of the maxillary left central and lateral incisors (Figs 14-1a to 14-1f).

Key Message

Injuries to the maxillary central incisors are approximately twice as frequent among children with increased overjet as in children with normal occlusion. Inadequate lip coverage results in threefold risk of tooth injury to maxillary incisors compared with children with complete lip coverage.[1]

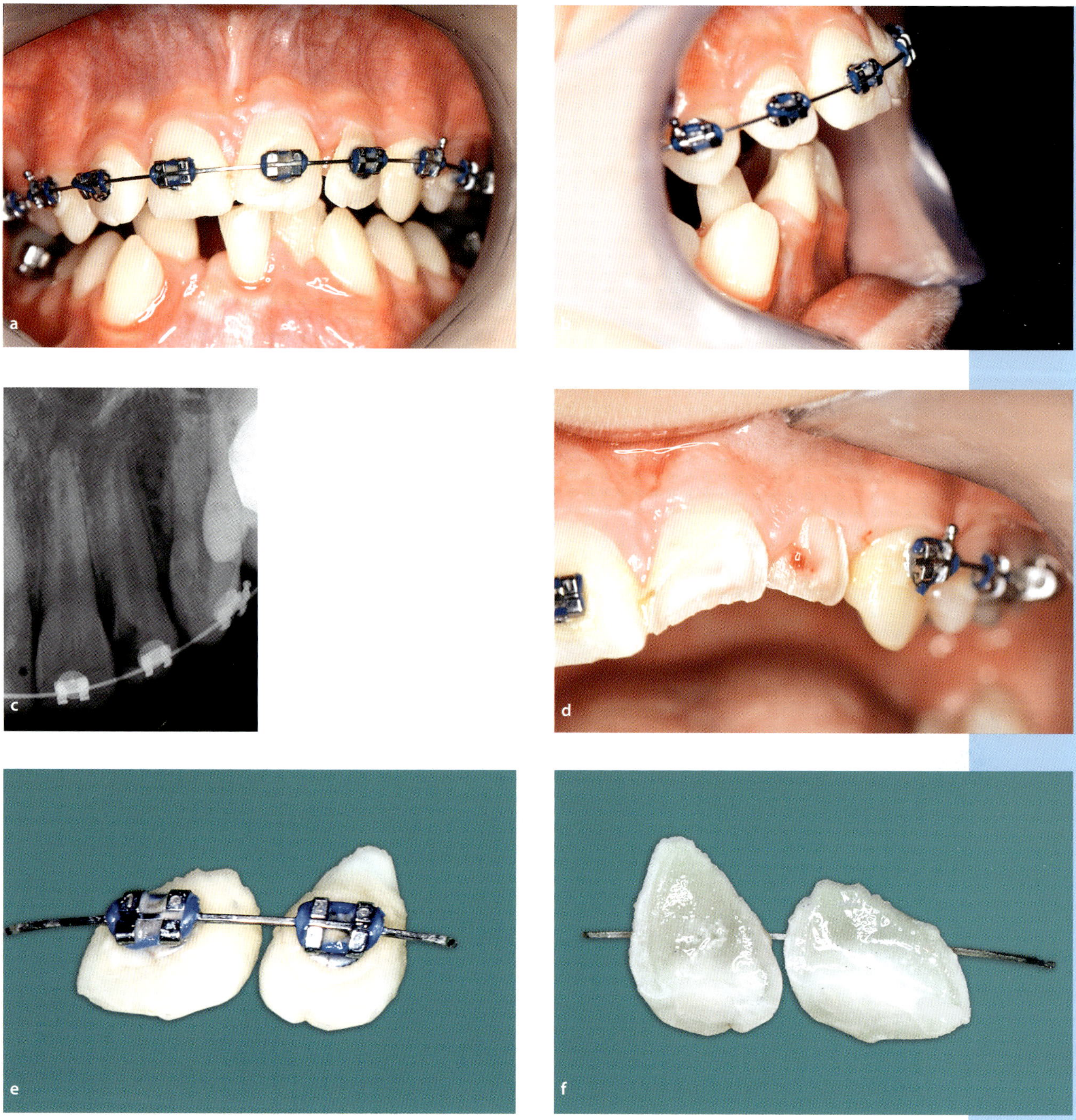

Fig. 14-1a–f Clinical findings after dental trauma: the impact to the chin was transferred to dental arches with vertical crown fractures of the maxillary left central and lateral incisors; the increased overjet and insufficient lip coverage were predisposing factors for crown injury. 14-1c Radiographic findings showed fracture lines in the crown area of both left maxillary incisors (21, 22). 14-1e, 14-1f After removal of the crown fragments of both incisors, 14-1d pulp exposure was evident in both the teeth.

CASE DESCRIPTION

History

Medical History
Simon was a healthy boy with no other illness.

Dental History
Simon was a regular attender at the dental office. On the day of his dental injury, all his teeth were sound or had minor filings. The main complaint was the fracture of the maxillary left central and lateral incisors (21, 22) and tooth sensitivity to thermal stimuli. There were no other injuries. There was no history of loss of consciousness, vomiting, or headache. Simon came for treatment 20 hours after the injury occurred. The full extent of the injury was established after removal of the orthodontic archwire, with the crown fragments. There was no increased mobility of teeth or sensitivity on percussion.

Oral Hygiene

Simon's oral hygiene used to be relatively good. After the injury, however, he was avoiding thorough toothbrushing, leading to visible dental plaque in the cervical region of the upper incisors and a slight colour change of the marginal gingiva. He was given instructions on oral hygiene maintenance and his mother was asked to supervise his toothbrushing.

Examination

The clinical examination revealed slight bruises on the skin under the chin and vertical fractures of enamel and dentin of the two left maxillary incisors (21, 22) with pulpal involvement. The labial crown fragments were still attached to the orthodontic brackets and archwire. In order to establish a proper diagnosis, it was necessary to remove the orthodontic wire. The wire was cut with the help of a high-speed diamond bur between the two central incisors (11, 21) and between the lateral incisor and the canine (22, 23) (Fig. 14-1a). On removal of the fractured segments it was seen that the pulp of the central incisor was very slightly exposed while the lateral incisor had a pulp exposure greater than 3 mm in diameter. The exposed pulps looked healthy.

Additional Investigations

Radiographs were taken of all the maxillary incisors to establish the apical status of the teeth and the presence/absence of root fractures. There were no visible root fractures or pathology around the affected teeth. The apices of the roots of both teeth were closed as expected at this age (usually 3 years after tooth eruption, ie, after 9 and 10 years, respectively, for the central and lateral incisors).

TREATMENT AIM

The aims of the treatment were:

- to maintain pulp vitality of both incisors by stimulating deposition of reparative or tertiary dentin and the formation of a dentinal bridge beneath the pulp exposure. This was to be achieved by pulp capping or by partial or Cvek pulpotomy[2–4]
- restore the lost crown tissue with a resin composite.

TREATMENT OPTIONS

Definitive

- Pulp treatment with preservation of pulp vitality with dentin bridge formation at the exposure site.
- Resin composite restoration of the fractured permanent central and lateral incisors.

Alternatives

- Endodontic treatment with root canal filling if pulp vitality was not maintained.
- Ceramic laminate veneers for the restoration of the buccal surfaces of both injured incisors.

Rationale

The exposed pulp tissue in complicated crown fractures shows an immediate inflammatory response. The surface of the pulp is covered by a layer of fibrin. Inflammatory changes do not involve more than about 2 mm depth of pulp tissue.[4,5] This observation is important for the therapeutic approach and treatment planning. Even if left untreated, traumatically exposed pulp remains vital for long periods of time. A few days after pulp exposure, hyperplasia of pulp tissue is a typical reaction. The superficial inflammation does not extend more than 2 mm from the exposure site.[4]

The exposed dental pulp can be treated by pulp capping, partial pulpotomy, complete pulpotomy, or pulpal extirpation.[4,6] The maturity of the tooth and the condition of the apex formation are important factors in the choice of treatment. The pulp vitality should be particularly maintained in young permanent teeth with incomplete root formation. If the tooth has had concomitant luxation injury, the pulp circulation could be additionally compromised. The chance for such complications is lower in immature teeth with an open apex.

When the pulp exposure is small (smaller than 1.5 mm in diameter) pulp capping is recommended. The recommended capping agents are hard-setting calcium hydroxide and mineral trioxide aggregate (MTA). A partial Cvek pulpotomy should be used for large pulp exposures (larger than 1.5 mm in diameter) with calcium hydroxide or MTA as dressing agents for the exposed pulp.

> ***Key Message***
> *The aim of treatment of permanent teeth with traumatic pulp exposure is preservation of pulp vitality and formation of a hard tissue barrier at the site of the pulp exposure.*

TREATMENT AND FOLLOW-UP

Treatment

The central incisor (21) with the small pulp exposure was treated by direct pulp capping, and the lateral incisor (22) with a partial pulpotomy (Figs 14-2a to 14-2d).

> ***Key Message***
> *Vital pulp therapy in permanent teeth has high success rates.*
>
> *Pulp capping as a simple method should be used when the pulp shows a small exposure (less than 1.5 mm in diameter) and is relatively uninflamed.*
>
> *The alternative method for greater pulp exposures and more infected pulps is a partial or Cvek pulpotomy. Although it requires more time to perform, it gives more predictable results with high success rates.*

Posttreatment Evaluation/Follow-up

Simon's teeth were monitored clinically (no history of pain or swelling), and checked for continued vitality.

Pulp vitality testing (electrical pulp testing, thermal testing), palpation, and percussion should be performed at 4 weeks, 8 weeks (Figs 14-3a, 14-3b), 3 months, 6 months, 1 year, and annually for a minimum of 3 years. Check radiographs should be taken after 2 months, 6 months, 1 year, and then annually for the next 3 years.[4]

After 2 months, the patient's incisors (21, 22) were restored with resin composite (Figs 14-4a, 14-4b). Radiographs taken after 2 years showed a hard tissue barrier at the site of pulp coverage and normal root formation (Figs 14-5a to 14-5d).

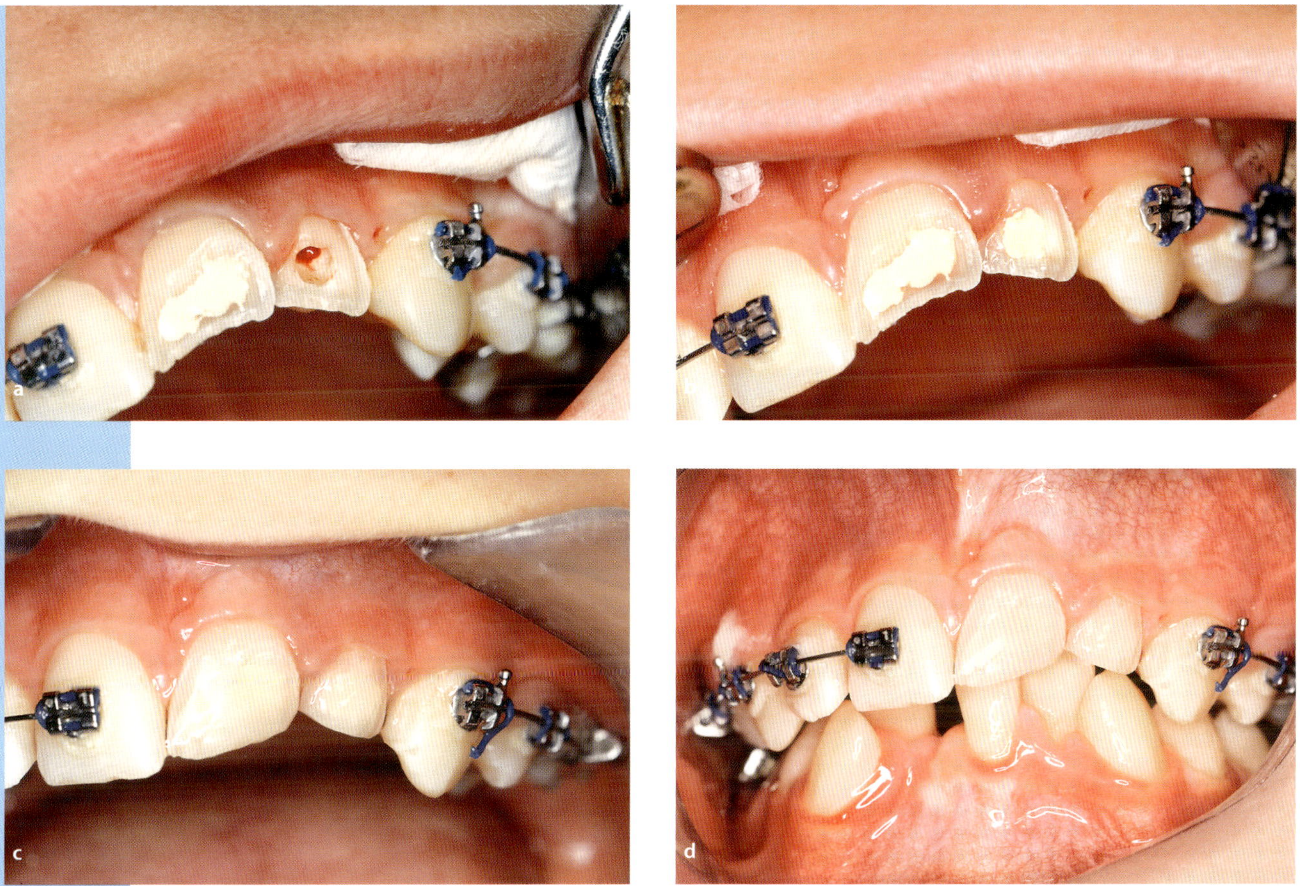

Fig. 14-2a–d Treatment by means of direct pulp capping in the maxillary left central incisor (21) involved 14-2a the use of calcium hydroxide (Dycal) and partial pulpotomy in the maxillary left lateral incisor (22). 14-2b After hemostasis, a hard-setting calcium hydroxide (Dycal) was used to cover the pulp tissue after pulpotomy. 14-2c, 14-2d Both teeth were acid-etched, washed, and dried and covered with temporary resin composite restorations for retention of the calcium hydroxide.

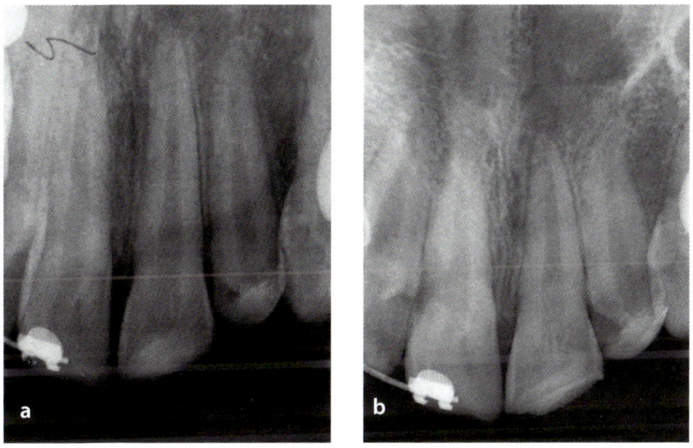

Fig. 14-3 Radiographic findings after 14-3a 2 months and 14-3b 6 months showing normal pulp healing without pathologic changes.

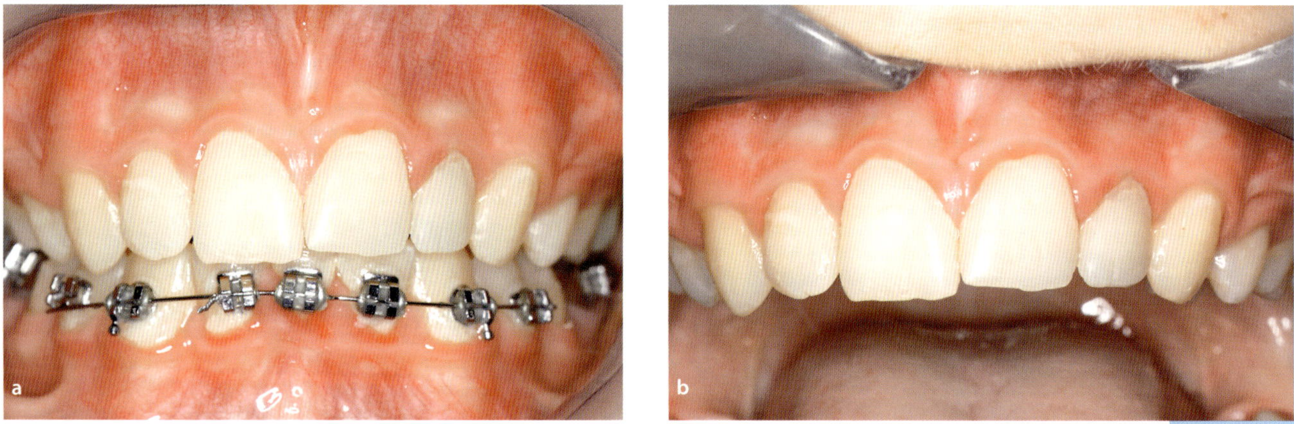

Fig. 14-4a,b Two months after pulp treatment, both incisors (21, 22) were restored with a hybrid resin composite.

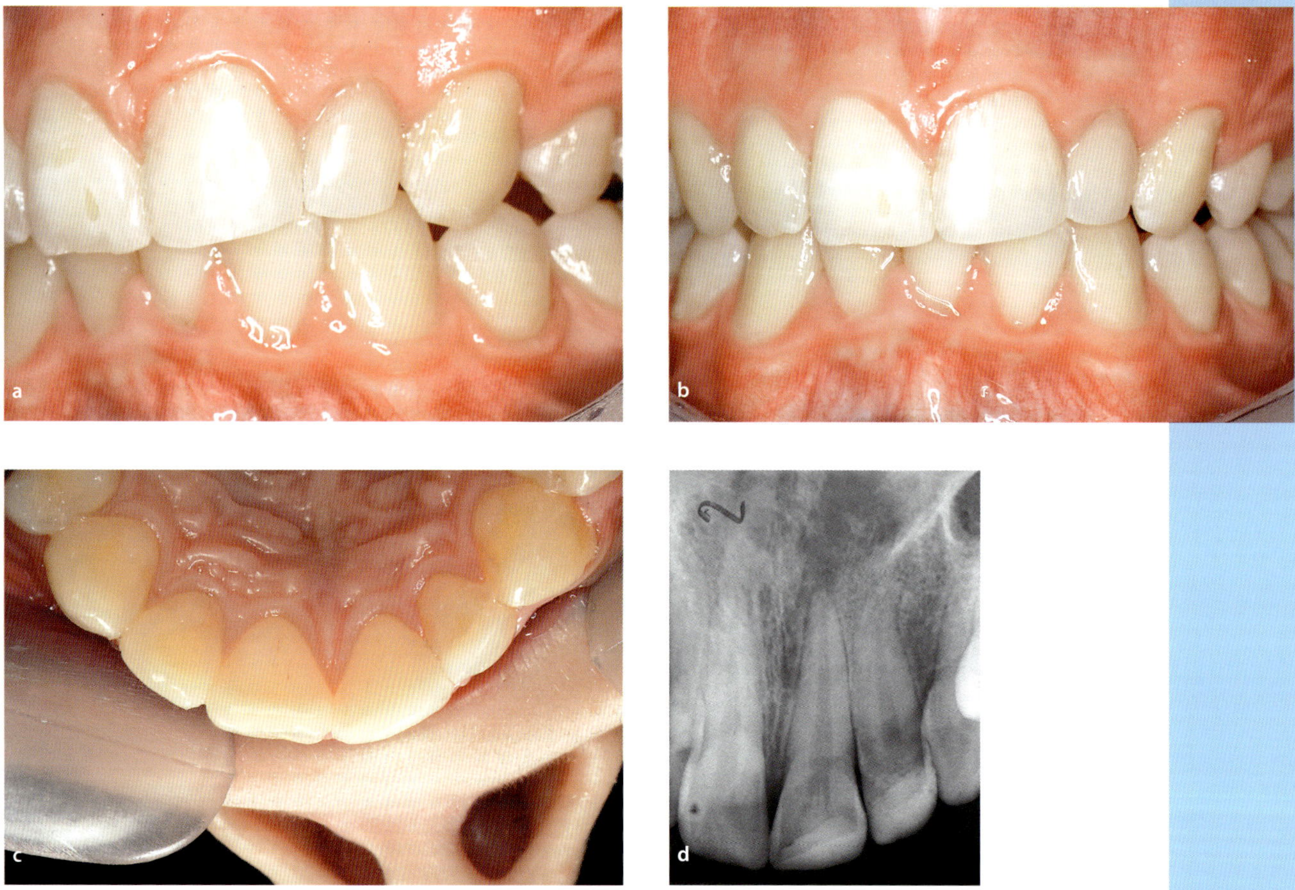

Fig. 14-5a–d A radiograph taken after 2 years shows the formation of a hard tissue barrier at the sites of the pulp coverage and normal root formation without pathologic changes.

DISCUSSION

Direct pulp capping is indicated when a small pulp exposure (up to 1.5 mm) is treated shortly after an injury (ie, within 24 hours after a trauma). Different agents have been proposed for pulp capping. The traditional material that is most widely used is calcium hydroxide. It provides repair of the pulp exposure site with hard tissue bridge deposition – what is considered to be a desirable and successful treatment. MTA is used as an alternative to calcium hydroxide for pulp capping and pulpotomies. Some studies have shown MTA to be superior to calcium hydroxide. Pulp capped with MTA exhibits less inflammation and a higher rate of dentin bridge formation.[7] Some studies have recommended pulp capping with dentin adhesive systems[8,9] but more recent research has shown that their use leads to the formation of pulp microabscesses, intense chronic inflammation of the pulp, and pulp necrosis.[10]

The pulpal wound is washed with saline and covered with soft or hard-setting calcium hydroxide. If a soft calcium hydroxide paste is used, the exposed dentin should be protected with glass-ionomer cement before crown restoration. The aim is to protect vital pulp from bacteria and other irritants, and to promote pulp healing and hard tissue formation at the exposure site. The surrounding exposed dentinal tubules should also be sealed to protect the pulp from bacterial penetration. It is suggested to apply dentin bonding agents after covering exposed pulp. Therefore, the dentinal margins close to enamel are left uncovered to provide a surface for the dentin bonding agent to bond to, before placing a composite restoration.

After pulp capping, a provisional resin composite restoration is placed to keep the calcium hydroxide at the site of pulp exposure and to prevent microleakage around the dressing material.

Partial pulpotomy (Cvek pulpotomy) is the procedure of removal of the superficial infected layer of pulp to the level of healthy coronal pulp. It is indicated for the immature teeth with an open apex as well as for mature teeth with a closed apex. The rationale for Cvek pulpotomy is that by removing the infected and inflamed pulp tissue and covering the underlying healthy tissue with the pulpotomy agent, a hard tissue barrier will form at the exposure site. After traumatic pulp exposure only superficial pulp contamination occurs. Histologic investigations show that even after 8 days only a superficial pulp layer (up to 1–1.5 mm) becomes infected while the pulp towards the apex remains vital and non-infected.

The technique of shallow pulpotomy for treatment of traumatized teeth with a pulp exposure was developed in Sweden by Miomir Cvek (1978). Crown fractures with pulp involvement and an exposed pulp require pulp preservation. The time between injury and treatment and size of the pulp exposure are not critical for the success of this procedure. It has highly predictable results and high rates of clinical success (about 95%).[4,5,11,12]

If a partial pulpotomy is indicated, the tooth has to be anesthetized and isolated. The surface pulp layer is usually removed to a depth of up to 2 mm using sterile, abrasive diamond burs at high speed with water cooling. After the bleeding has ceased the wound at the amputation site is covered by calcium hydroxide or by MTA as a standard procedure.[4,6] The resin composite restoration is then placed to seal the tooth.

Immature permanent teeth with incomplete roots have a better chance for pulp preservation, but a completed root is not a contraindication for a partial pulpotomy.[4,13]

Complete pulpotomy (cervical pulpotomy) is the removal of the coronal pulp tissue and the placement of a dressing material (calcium hydroxide or MTA) on the surface of the radicular pulp tissue. This procedure will preserve the vitality of the root pulp and allows full root development in permanent immature teeth. A complete endodontic procedure will follow only if the root canal is required for the retention of a root post for prosthetic treatment. The success rate is lower than for a partial pulpotomy and ranges from 90% at 6 months to 78% at 12 months.[3]

SUMMARY

In management of complicated crown fractures, retention of capping material and prevention of microleakage are crucial factors. Microleakage and bacterial penetration are the main causes of treatment failure, pulpal inflammation, and necrosis. Use of dentin bonding systems can provide better marginal seal. Partial pulpotomy could be considered the method of choice for treatment of traumatically exposed pulp because it gives highly predictable results with success rates ranging from 94% to 100%.[4,5,14] The high rate of success for partial pulpotomy is considered to be related to the efficient sealing of the pulp exposure by dressing and restorative materials such as glass ionomer or dentin adhesives with resin composites.

Key Message
All methods of vital pulp therapy give more predictable results when applied to teeth with traumatic pulp exposure than in teeth with carious pulp exposure.

REFERENCES

1. Andreasen JO, Andreasen FM, Andersson L (eds) Textbook and Color Atlas of Traumatic Injuries to the Teeth, 4th edn. Copenhagen: Blackwell Munksgaard, 2007.
2. Olsburgh S, Krejci I. Pulp response to traumatic crown fractures. Endodontic Topics 2003;5:26–40.
3. Swift EJ Jr, Trope M, Ritter AV. Vital pulp therapy for the mature tooth – can it work? Endodontic Topics 2003;5:49–56.
4. Cvek M. Endodontic management and the use of calcium hydroxide in traumatized permanent teeth. In: Andreasen JO, Andreasen FM, Andersson L (eds) Textbook and Color Atlas of Traumatic Injuries to the Teeth, 4th edn. Copenhagen: Blackwell Munksgaard, 2007:598–657.
5. Cvek M. A clinical report on partial pulpotomy and capping with calcium hydroxide in permanent incisors with complicated crow fracture. J Endod 1978;4:232–237.
6. American Academy of Pediatric Dentistry. Guideline on pulp therapy for primary and young permanent teeth. Pediatr Dent 2007;29(suppl.):163–167.
7. Faraco IM Jr, Holland R. Response of the pulp of dogs to capping with mineral trioxide aggregate or a calcium hydroxide cement. Dent Traumatol 2001;17:163–166.
8. Heitmann T, Unterbrink G. Direct pulp capping with a dentinal adhesive resin system: a pilot study. Quintessence Int 1995;26:765–770.
9. Schuurs AHB, Gruythuysen RJM, Wesselink PR. Pulp capping with adhesive resin-based composite vs. calcium hydroxide: a review. Endod Dent Traumatol 2000;16:240–250.
10. Mestrener SR, Holland R, Dezan E Jr. Influence of age on the behavior of dental pulp of dog teeth after capping with an adhesive system or calcium hydroxide. Dent Traumatol 2003;19:255–261.
11. Olsburgh S, Jakoby T, Krejci I. Crown fractures in the permanent dentition: pulpal and restorative considerations. Dent Traumatol 2002;18:103–115.
12. American Academy of Pediatric Dentistry. Guideline on management of acute dental trauma. Pediatr Dent 2007;29(suppl.):168–176.
13. Cvek M, Lundberg M. Histological appearance of pulps after exposure by a crown fracture, partial pulpotomy, and clinical diagnosis of healing. J Endod 1983;9:8–11.
14. Fuks AB, Cosack A, Klein H, Eidelman E. Partial pulpotomy as a treatment alternative for exposed pulps in crown-fractured permanent incisors. Endod Dent Traumatol 1987;3:100–102.

15 Traumatic Bone Cyst

Anna Lena Sundell

Key words: traumatic bone cyst, simple bone cyst, solitary bone cyst, extravasation cyst, unicameral bone cyst, progressive bone cavity

Age category: 10–20 years

Definition

Traumatic bone cyst is an unusual osteolytic process in bone that seldom gives rise to symptoms. As a result, this type of cyst is often first detected at routine radiographic examinations. The etiology and pathogenesis are still uncertain, which is reflected by the variety of synonyms used (see key words above) (Figs 15-1a to 15-1d).

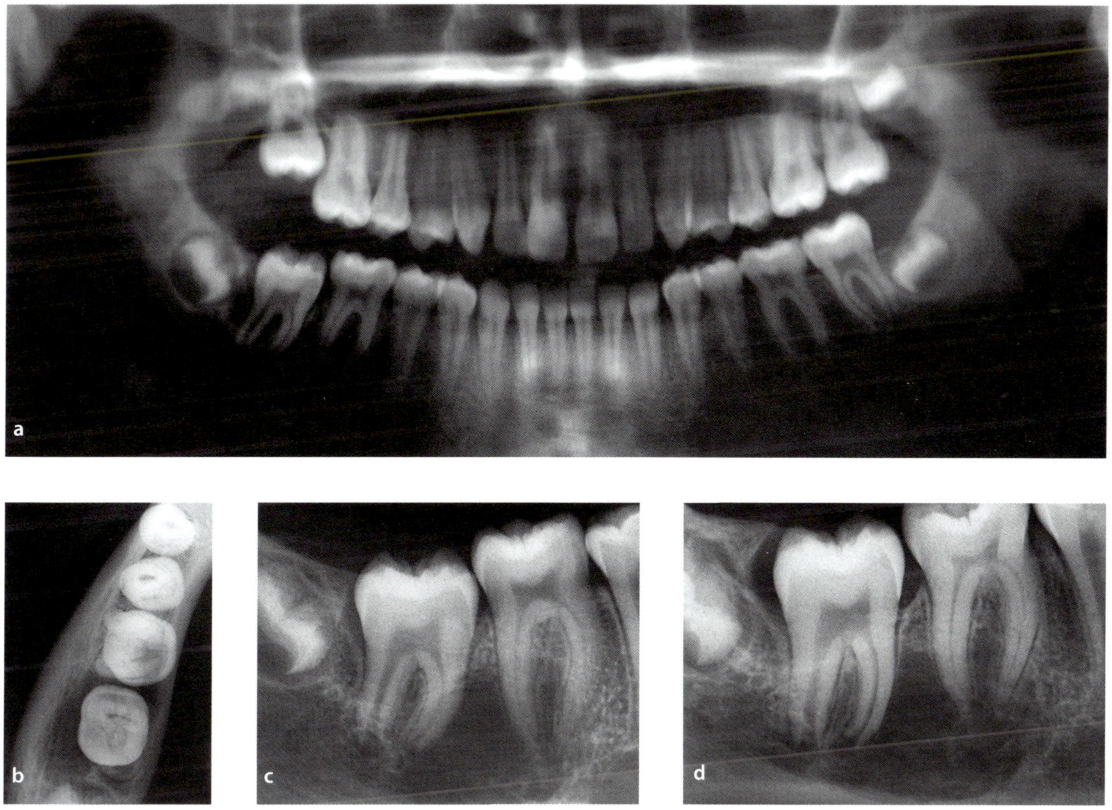

Fig. 15-1a–d A 14-year-old patient with traumatic bone cyst. A defined radiolucent area is seen in the region of the mandibular right first and second molars (46, 47).

THE PROBLEM

The patient has no clinical symptoms related to her teeth or mouth. A radiolucent lesion was seen on routine oral radiographic examination.

CASE DESCRIPTION

History

Medical History
ASA I. Joan was a healthy 14-year-old girl, who had been adopted from Colombia when she was 5 years old. There was little information about her early years of life and there was no known history of trauma to the face.

Dental History
Joan had never had any decay and, consequently, she had no experience of invasive dental treatment. She saw her dentist once a year for routine examination of the oral cavity. She was referred to the department of pediatric dentistry after her dentist found a radiolucent area in the region of the mandibular right first and second molars (46, 47). The cyst was an occasional finding on the panoramic radiograph taken as part of the radiologic examination performed prior to treatment planning for the patient's proclined incisors and median diastema.

Oral Hygiene

Oral hygiene was good. Joan brushed her teeth twice a day with a fluoridated dentifrice.

Examination

Intraoral examination did not reveal any pathologic conditions concerning the oral mucosa or the teeth. The examination showed proclined maxillary incisors with a median diastema.

Additional Investigations

The panoramic radiograph shows a radiolucent area in the region of the mandibular right first and second molars (46, 47). Periapical and segmental occlusal radiographs were taken to visualize the margins of the lesion. The radiolucency was partly distinct and was about 2.5 cm x 1 cm in size. It was located between the mandibular right first and second molars, extending to the buccal side of the mandibular second molar. The mesial part of the lesion was distinct, while the distal part was more diffusely defined. In the distal part of the lesion multilocular areas were also visible. The lesion had a certain radiopacity on its medial/inferior aspect. The teeth involved with the lesion were vital on electrical pulp testing.

DIAGNOSIS AND TREATMENT AIM

The aim of the treatment was surgical intervention, first to confirm the clinical diagnosis of traumatic bone cyst and second to carry out the treatment in order to achieve complete healing.

> ***Key Message***
> *Complete healing is important as traumatic bone cysts may recur if complete healing is not acheived.*

TREATMENT OPTIONS

Definitive

- Exploratory surgery with curettage.

Alternatives

- Aspiration of fluid from the cyst.

Rationale

The therapy of choice was exploratory surgery with curettage. This treatment would initiate osteoblastic activity by attracting mesenchymal cells in the blood to the cyst site, which differentiate into cells with osteogenetic potential.[1] In some cases, complete regression has been achieved by aspiration of the fluid of the cyst.[2] In order to confirm the diagnosis, samples of fluid and material from the curettage should be sent for histologic examination.

Traumatic bone cysts may recur unless complete healing is achieved.[1,3,4] After the surgical intervention, the area of the cyst should therefore be followed up clinically and radiographically until the lesion has completely healed.

> ***Key Message***
> *If there is the slightest risk of discovering a pathologic process during the surgery, diagnostic samples should be taken for histologic examination.*

TREATMENT AND FOLLOW-UP

Treatment

It was decided to surgically explore the lesion along with curettage. Surgery was performed under general anesthesia since the patient had no previous experience of dental treatment. A mucogingival flap was raised and the area of bone destruction exposed. The covering buccal bone was hollow and blood vessels penetrating the cortical bone could be seen. Bone was removed under water cooling and the lesion inspected. It seemed to be empty with no epithelial or connective tissue lining. Small parts of bone were removed and sent for histologic examination. This examination revealed normally formed bone, a common finding in traumatic bone cysts.

Posttreatment Evaluation/Follow-up

The prognosis was good. The traumatic bone cyst was completely healed at the final checkup, 6 years after the exploratory surgery. No more checkups on a regular basis were needed concerning this area (Figs 15-2a, 15-2b).

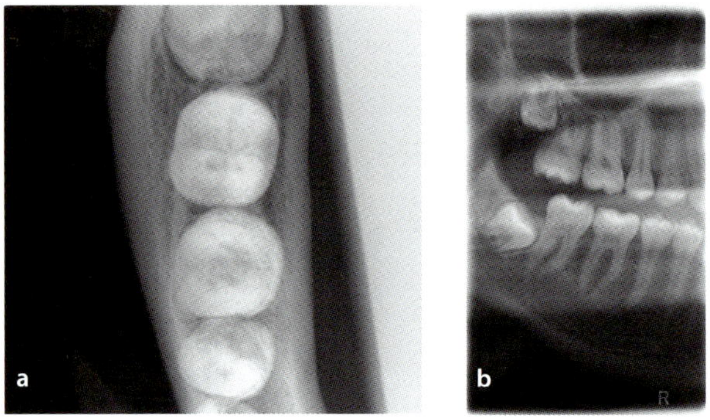

Fig. 15-2a,b Six-year checkup. Complete healing of the area of the bone cyst is seen.

DISCUSSION

Traumatic bone cyst was reported in the literature for the first time in 1929.[1–5] It is an unusual osteolytic process that seldom gives rise to any symptoms. That is one reason why this type of cyst is often detected coincidentally at routine radiographic examination. Nowadays, radiographic examinations involving panoramic radiographs are common in treatment planning within dentistry. This explains why more traumatic bone cysts are found today and it is reasonable to believe that traumatic bone cysts probably are more common than previously thought. The cysts are often detected between the ages of 10 and 20 years,[5–7] but they are seldom found in adults. It has therefore been speculated that traumatic bone cysts disappear spontaneously since they otherwise would have been as common in adults as in younger individuals.[8]

Hansen[6] has shown that these cysts are equally common in girls and boys. Earlier studies have reported a higher prevalence in men. In older patients, an increased prevalence has been seen in dark-skinned women.[7] The majority of traumatic bone cysts in the jaws are found in the mandible and often in the posterior part where they probably begin to develop above the mandibular canal,[6] which was also the situation in the present patient's case. Bone cysts can also occur in other parts of the body, most commonly in the humerus or the femur.

Radiographic examination of a traumatic bone cyst will reveal either a unilocular or a multilocular, well-delineated radiolucency. If teeth are involved, scalloped cyst margins will be seen that extend between the roots of the teeth. The lamina dura is always intact and the teeth are seldom displaced.[6] Sometimes there may be thinning of the cortical bone with osseous expansion.[1,2,9,10] Teeth in and around the affected area are often vital.[6,10,11]

The cavity lacks an epithelial lining, which is one of the criteria for diagnosis. Histologic examination may show a thin connective tissue membrane lining the cavity, but no other significant features will be seen.[1,4,10] The bone around the cyst is normal. The cavity is either empty or filled with fluid that contains fragments of connective tissue, blood or degenerated products of blood and granulation tissue. The color of the fluid varies from yellow-green to red-brown depending on contents. In the present case, the lesion was empty and had no epithelial lining.

The origin of traumatic bone cysts is unknown, but the most accepted explanation is trauma-initiated intramedullary arterial bleeding that results in degeneration of the trabecular bone followed by resorption.[2,3,6,7,10] Lack of healing is due to a blood clot that is not organized in the usual way. Other probable reasons that have been described are: degeneration of benign neoplasms; focal low-grade chronic infection; local disturbance of bone growth which results in osteolysis; venous obstruction; as well as faulty calcium metabolism secondary to parathyroid disease.[3,7] History of trauma has been verified in about half of reported patients with traumatic bone cysts.[6] Our patient had no known history of trauma to her face.

The differential diagnoses of traumatic bone cysts are: odontogenic keratocysts, follicular cysts, ameloblastomas, odontogenic fibromas, and odontogenic myxomas.

- Odontogenic keratocysts and follicular cysts are, unlike traumatic bone cysts, lined with epithelium and often localized in connection with an unerupted tooth. These cysts can also displace and resorb nearby existing teeth and bone.

- An ameloblastoma is also located close to an unerupted tooth. It develops from various odontogenic epithelia. Clinically and radiographically it is difficult to separate ameloblastomas from traumatic bone cysts.
- Odontogenic myxomas can displace and resorb adjacent teeth. Radiographically, the distal part is often calcified, which is not the case in traumatic bone cysts. Both odontogenic myxomas and odontogenic fibromas contain mesenchymal soft tissue from the dental papilla and dental bud. Radiographically, fibromas and traumatic bone cysts look similar.

REFERENCES

1. Cowan CG. Traumatic bone cysts of the jaws and their presentation. Int J Oral Surg 1980;9:287–291.
2. Chapman PJ, Romaniuk K. Traumatic bone cyst of the mandible; regression following aspiration. Int J Oral Surg 1985;14:290–294.
3. Breen GH, Addante R. A recurrent traumatic bone cyst: report of case. ASDC J Dent Child 1994;61:141–145.
4. Friedrichsen SW. Long-term progression of a traumatic bone cyst. A case report. Oral Surg Oral Med Oral Pathol 1993;76:421–424.
5. Hansen LS, Sapone J, Sproat RC. Traumatic bone cysts of jaws. Oral Surg Oral Med Oral Pathol 1974;37:899–910.
6. Pindborg JJ, Hjørting-Hansen E. Atlas of Diseases of the Jaws. Copenhagen: Munksgaard, 1974.
7. Oliveira DT, Hoshi AT, dos Reis OP. Clinical management of traumatic bone cyst in children: a case report. J Clin Pediatr Dent 2000;24: 107–110.
8. Dellinger TM, Holder R, Livingston HM, Hill WJ. Alternative treatments for a traumatic bone cyst: a longitudinal case report. Quintessence Int 1998;29:497–502.
9. Scholl RJ, Kellett HM, Neumann DP, Lurie AG. Cysts and cystic lesions of the mandible: clinical and radiologic-histopathologic review. Radiographics 1999;19:1107–1124.
10. Shafer H, Hine MK, Levy BM. A Textbook of Oral Pathology. Philadelphia: WB Saunders Company, 1983.
11. Neves A, Migliari DA, Sugaya NN, de Sousa SO. Traumatic bone cyst: report of two cases and review of the literature. Gen Dent 2001;49: 291–295, quiz 6–7.

16

Pulp Therapy in the Primary Molars

Monty Duggal

Key words: ferric sulfate, pulpotomy, pulpectomy, coronal pulp, radicular pulp

Age category: 4–7 years

Definitions

Pulpotomy is the procedure of removing the coronal part of the pulp tissue, inflamed as a result of deep caries, and maintenance of the vital radicular pulp tissue. Usually a medicament such as ferric sulfate is applied to achieve hemostasis before a coronal restoration is placed. Formocresol is also still widely used, though its mode of action is "fixation" rather than hemostasis. *Pulpectomy* is a procedure of extirpating the entire inflamed or infected pulp, both from the pulp chamber and the root canals and filling the root canals with a suitable material, usually zinc oxide based, to maintain the primary tooth in a non-infected state.

THE PROBLEM

Rory (4½ years old), was first seen in April 2005 when he presented as an emergency patient at Leeds Dental Institute with acute pain in the lower right quadrant and occasional pain in the upper left one. The pain in the lower right quadrant was severe and made him wake up at night and cry. The pain in the upper left quadrant started when he had anything to eat or drink and then gradually subsided, but never woke him up at night. He also complained that food got wedged between his upper left back teeth and this also gave him discomfort. His regular dentist never restored these teeth as he felt that these were only "baby" teeth and did not need to be restored. As an emergency procedure we extracted the mandibular right primary second molar (85) on this emergency visit for relief of pain, using local analgesia.

CASE DESCRIPTION

History

Medical History

Rory is a fit and healthy child with no allergies or disabilities. There was no history of previous hospital admissions.

Dental History

There was a history of facial swelling related to an abscessed mandibular right second primary molar (85) which was managed initially by extraction carried out in an emergency appointment and the patient was given a further appointment for more comprehensive care. He attended with his mother and was very cooperative. Rory's mother reported a loss of his maxillary anterior primary tooth following trauma. A few months later, a "funny shaped" tooth erupted in its place. His mother was not concerned at all and thought that the newly erupted tooth was the permanent successor. But now the main concern was the pain on the upper left side which sometimes made the patient cry.

Oral Hygiene

Rory brushed his teeth twice daily (morning and night) with a children's toothpaste with no supervision. His oral hygiene was fair but needed improvement.

Examination

On examination, the patient had clinically obvious carious lesions in the maxillary left primary first and second molars (64, 65). The maxillary left primary second molar was slightly tender to gentle percussion. Other minimal caries was observed in the occlusal surfaces of teeth as charted. The mandibular right primary second molar (85) had been extracted on a previous visit due to severe pain. There was also a mesiodens present in the upper anterior region (Figs 16-1a to 16-1c).

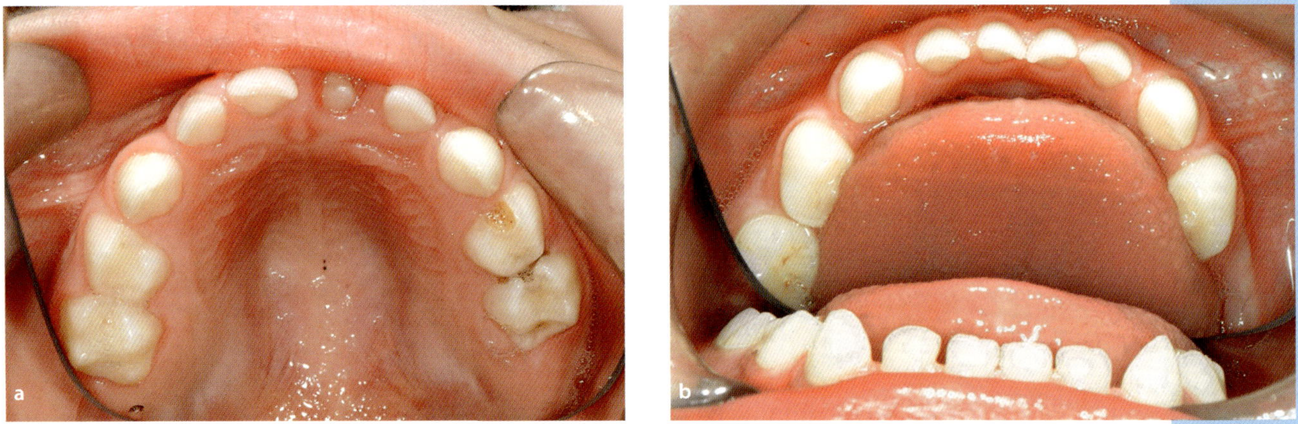

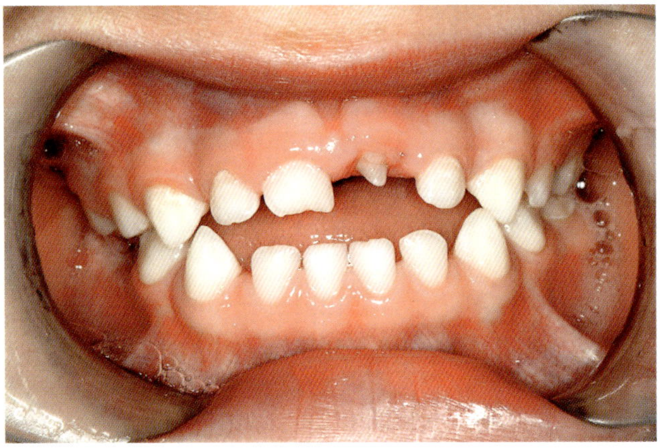

Fig. 16-1a–c Intraoral photographs showing caries in the maxillary left primary first and second molars (64, 65). Note that the mandibular right primary second molar (85) had previously been extracted, and the maxillary left primary central incisor (61) had been lost due to trauma on a previous occasion. Also note the conical mesiodens in the upper anterior region.

Additional Investigations

Panoramic and bitewing radiographs were taken (Fig. 16-2). The radiographs showed the following:

- all permanent teeth (except third molars) present and normally developed
- peg-shaped (mesiodens) supernumerary erupted in position of the maxillary left primary central incisor (61)
- rotated maxillary left central incisor (21)
- mandibular right primary second molar – gross caries, furcal pathology (extracted already)
- maxillary left primary second molar – proximal caries (mesial)
- maxillary left primary first molar – mesial caries with temporary dressing.

DIAGNOSIS

The diagnosis most relevant to this chapter relates to the upper left first and second primary molars (64, 65). It was noted that the marginal ridge of both molars was broken down with at least half of the intercuspal distance from the buccal to the palatal cusp involved in the carious process. This is

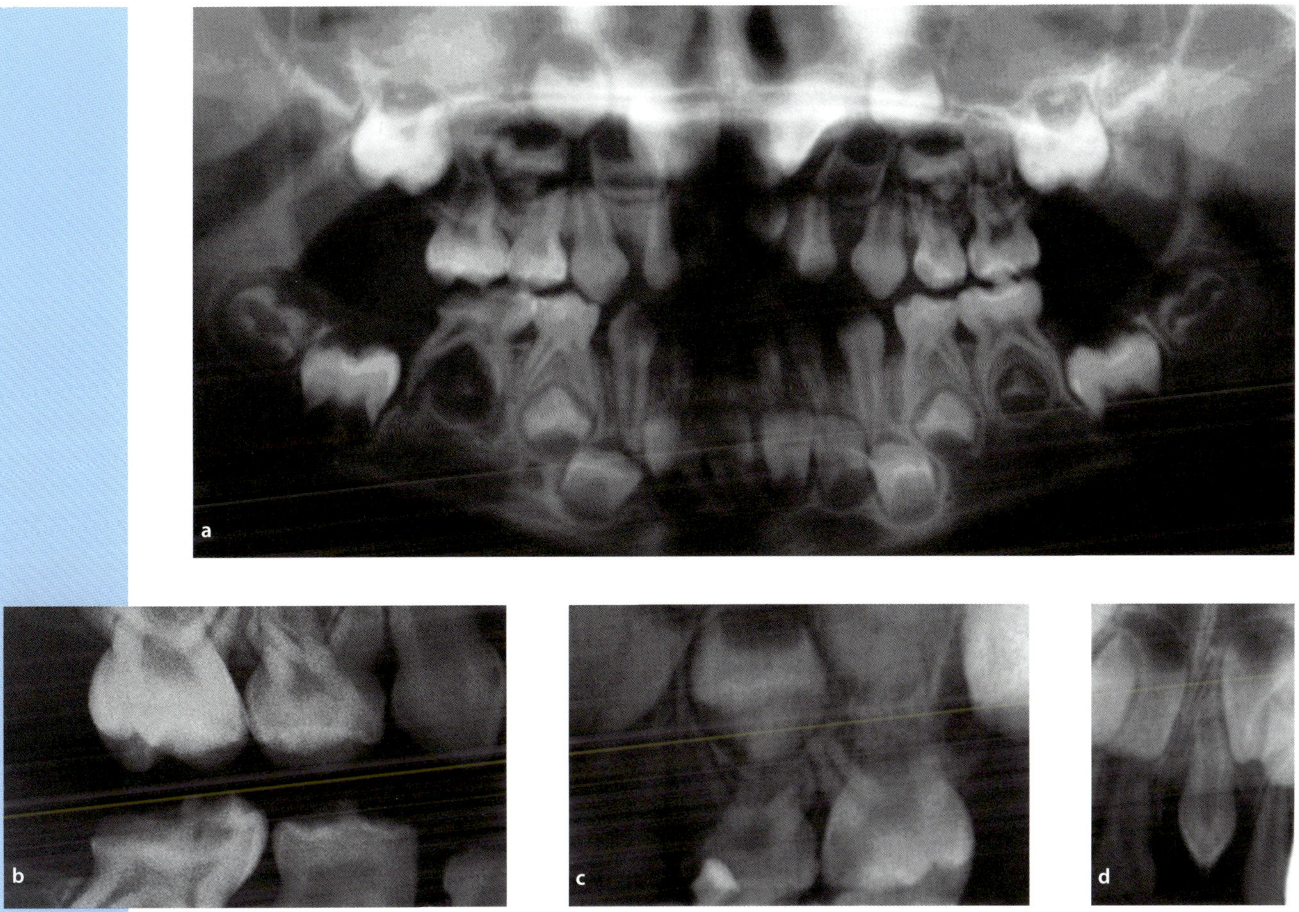

Fig. 16-2 Panoramic radiograph (16-2a), left and right bitewings (16-2b, 16-2c), and periapical radiograph (16-2d).

usually an indication of possible pulpal involvement and suggests that pulp might already be in a state of inflammation. Also, as the maxillary left primary second molar was tender to gentle percussion it was diagnosed as having either irreversible pulpitis and/or mild periapical periodontitis.

TREATMENT AIM

The aim of the treatment for this child was to manage the pulp pathology as a result of extensive caries in some primary molars.

TREATMENT OPTIONS

Definitive

It was decided to undertake comprehensive care using local analgesia for this patient. In addition to other restorative and preventive care and the management of the mesiodens that the patient required, for the purposes of this chapter emphasis will be placed on the pulp therapy carried out on the maxillary left primary first and second molars (64, 65). The treatment plan was:

- maxillary left primary first molar – vital pulpotomy with ferric sulfate and stainless steel crown
- maxillary left primary second molar – pulpectomy with Vitapex (Vitapex, New Dental Chemical Products, Tokyo) as root canal filling material and stainless steel crown.

Alternatives

It would have been possible to carry out the coronal restoration of both the maxillary left primary first and second molars (64, 65) using either amalgam or plastic restorations in the form of either resin composite or glass-ionomer cements. However, this was not done for two reasons. First, it was clear that pulp therapy was required on both the teeth, and these restorations do not provide as good a coronal seal as stainless steel crowns, and the chances of reinfection of the pulp due to a failing or leaking coronal restoration are high. Second, it is clear from the literature that plastic restorative materials do not perform as well as stainless steel crowns for restoration of proximal lesions.

Rationale

It is often difficult for clinicians to diagnose the status of the pulp effectively at the time of restoration of the tooth, especially in those with medium-sized to large proximal lesions. It has been shown in the literature[1] that when the marginal ridge is clinically obviously broken down, the pulp is already inflamed and the inflammation has already engulfed the pulp horn even when there is no clinically detectable exposure of the pulp. Large proximal restorations without pulp therapy usually have poor outcomes. The removal of the inflamed pulp is justified in order to ensure that the patient does not develop an abscess in the future. It was therefore decided to undertake a pulpotomy in this case for the maxillary left first primary molar (64).

Formocresol has been used for many decades in pediatric dental practice and beyond doubt has been one of the most successful pulp medicaments. However, there are questions about the safety of the chemicals that constitute this therapeutic material, in particular formaldehyde and cresol. In a prospective randomized controlled trial comparing formocresol with ferric sulfate,[2] the only such well-conducted study, a comparable efficacy was reported for formocresol and ferric sulfate. A number of other studies, although not as well conducted, have led to the same conclusion. Ferric sulfate is available commercially as 15.5% Astringedent™ (Ultradent). On contact with blood, a ferric ion–protein complex is formed, and the membrane of this complex seals the cut vessels mechanically producing hemostasis and preventing blood clot formation. Given this body of evidence, we carried out the pulpotomy on the maxillary left primary first molar (64) using ferric sulfate.

The upper second primary molar (65) was tender to gentle percussion so it was decided that a pulpectomy was required for this tooth. In order to preserve primary teeth with any evidence of periapical or bifurcation infection, it is necessary to clean and fill the root canals with a suitable material which will resorb along with the roots of the primary teeth. In this case we used Vitapex™, which is a combination of iodoform and calcium hydroxide. The material is easy to apply, resorbs at a slightly faster rate than that of the roots with no detrimental effects, has no toxic effect on the permanent successor, and is radio-opaque.

Both the maxillary left primary first and second molars (64, 65) were restored with stainless steel crowns after ferric sulfate pulpotomy and a pulpectomy procedure, respectively. Many studies have shown that stainless steel crowns are the most effective restorations for primary molars. A strong argument for use of the stainless steel crown restoration is its cost-effectiveness based on its durability and longevity. Roberts and colleagues[3] reported a success rate of 97% over 7 years.

Key Message

A breakdown of marginal ridge of more than 50% usually indicates that the pulp is already inflamed and a pulpotomy is required before the coronal restoration of the tooth.

After pulp therapy, stainless steel crowns provide the most durable and long-lasting restoration of the teeth, which then seldom need to be replaced. In addition, stainless steel crowns also provide an excellent coronal seal, which protects the pulp treatment from further infection.

TREATMENT AND FOLLOW-UP

Treatment was provided over two visits using local analgesia.

Treatment: Visit 1

After administering the local anesthetic and applying a rubber dam, the maxillary left primary second molar (65) was accessed and all caries removed. Access was gained to the pulp chamber and the root canals for the removal of necrotic pulp tissue. The three canals identified were: palatal, mesiobuccal, and distobuccal. After thorough irrigation and debridement the canals were filled with Vitapex using a spiral root canal filler on a slow speed handpiece. A postoperative radiograph (see Fig. 16-3a below) showed that all the canals were filled adequately. It was decided to carry out the stainless steel restoration on the next visit as the child was getting a little tired.

Treatment: Visit 2

Local anesthetic and rubber dam were applied again. The maxillary left primary first molar (64) was accessed, caries removed and a vital pulpotomy performed after gaining access to the pulp chamber. Vital coronal pulp was removed with sharp excavators and ferric sulfate applied on the radicular tissue on a cotton pledget for 1 minute to achieve hemostasis. The pulp chamber was then filled with zinc oxide cement and both the maxillary left primary first and second molars (64, 65) restored with stainless steel crowns. A postoperative radiograph showed that the treatment was adequate (Fig. 16-3b) and the patient was discharged. Figures 16-4a–c show the completed restorations.

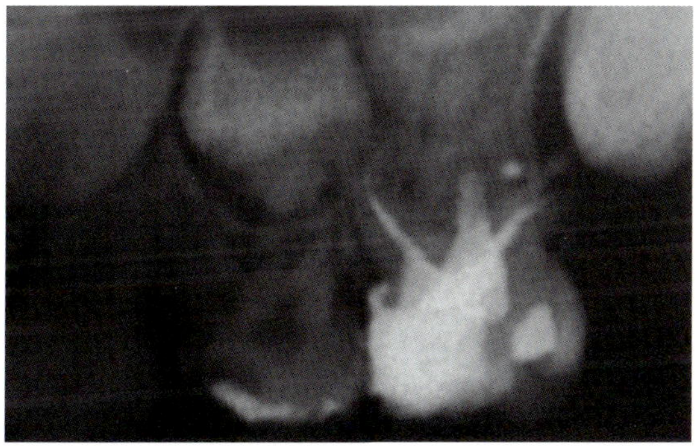

Fig. 16-3a Radiographs showing pulpectomy in the maxillary left primary second molar (65) before the stainless steel crown was placed.

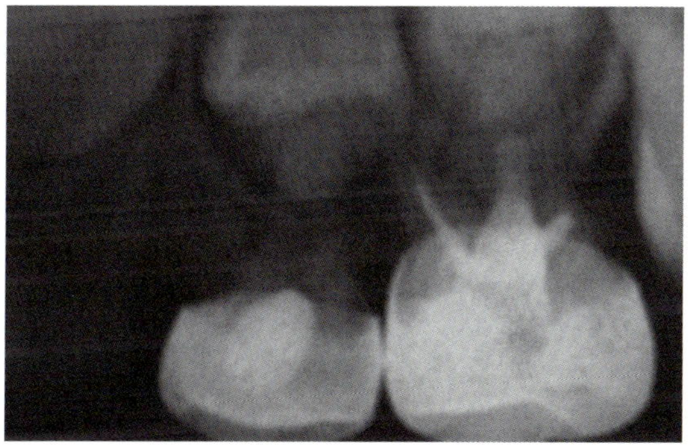

Fig. 16-3b Pulpotomy in the maxillary left primary first molar (64), and pulpectomy in the maxillary left primary second molar (65) after stainless steel crown restorations were placed.

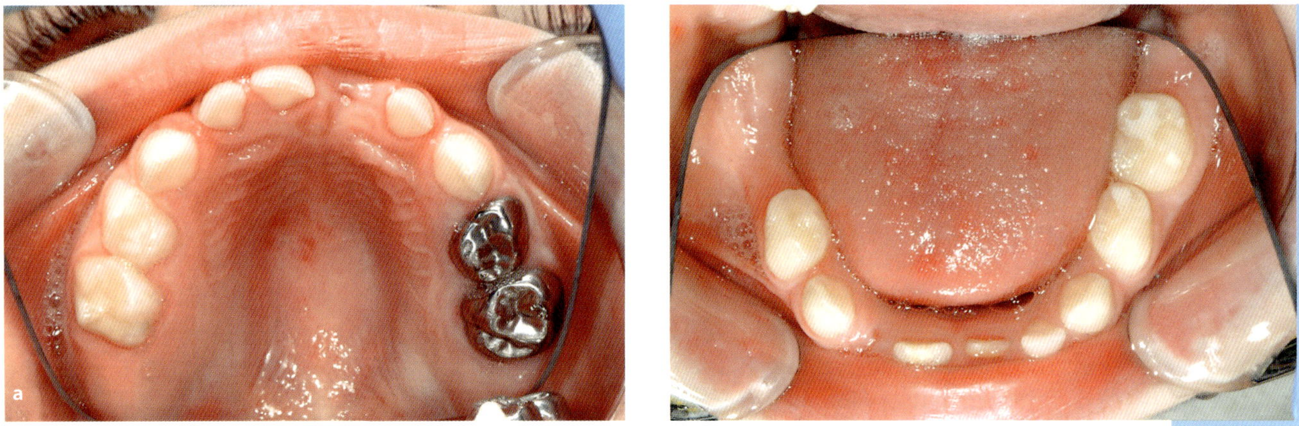

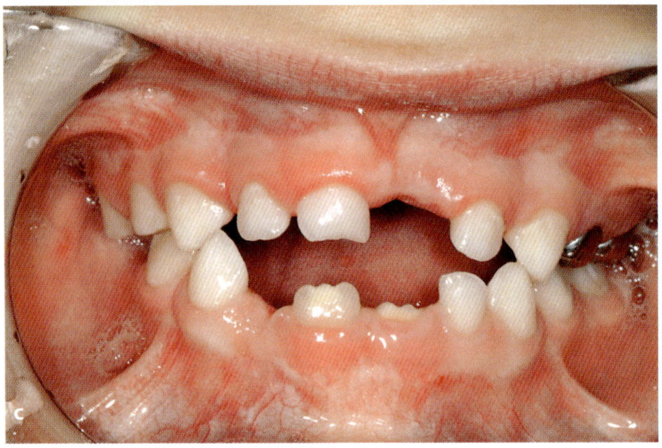

Fig. 16-4a–c Intraoral photographs showing completed restorations in the maxillary left primary first and second molars (64, 65). Note the excellent gingival adaptation of the crowns and also the excellent occlusion. 16-4c The other carious primary molars have been restored with minimal intervention technique and the mesiodens has also now been removed.

Posttreatment Evaluation/Follow-up

The patient remained free from pain or discomfort after 24 months of placement of the restorations (Figs 16-5a to 16-5c). The gingivae around the stainless steel crowns were not inflamed and were in excellent condition. Radiographic examination showed no furcation pathology and excellent bone condition around the pulp-treated teeth (Fig. 16-6). The oral hygiene had also improved. It was noted that the first permanent molars that had recently erupted showed signs of molar-incisor hypomineralization and the patient is now undergoing its management.

DISCUSSION

Children who still get caries deserve high-quality comprehensive treatment from dental professionals. The preventive approach is important, but in many patients restorative intervention is required. When restorations need to be done, care should be taken to use techniques and materials that do not need to be replaced or the treatment done repetitiously. Repetitious treatment has implications for the child's behavior. The approach shown in this case is one such high-quality approach. Restorations as have been placed should now last for the lifetime of the primary molars. Also, good quality care as provided here with a suitable behavior management technique gives a positive dental experience to the child and family and contributes to a better attitude to dental health in the long term.

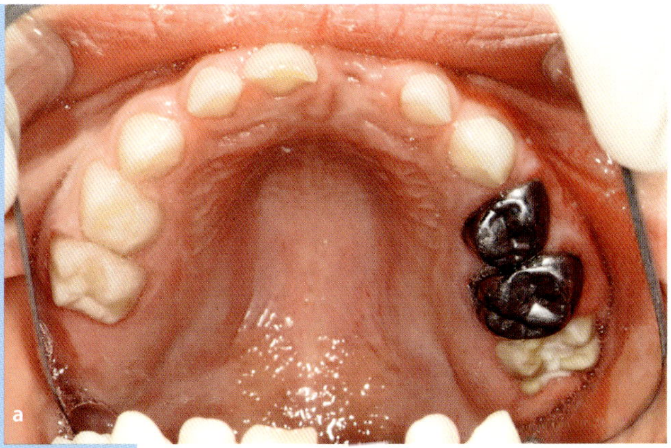

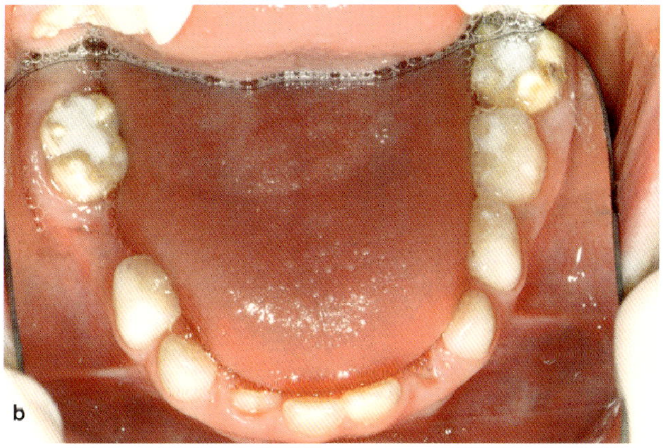

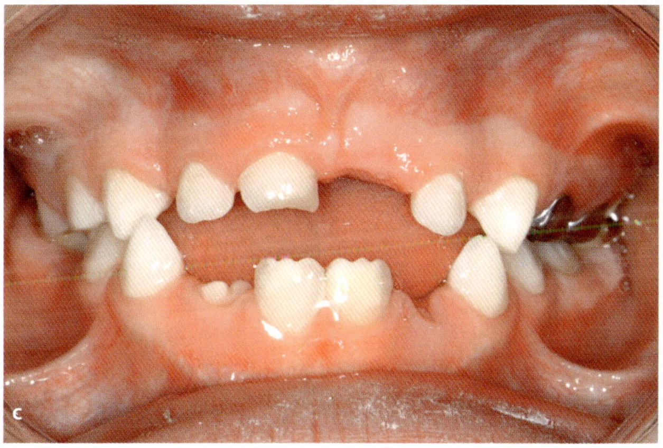

Fig. 16-5a–c Intraoral photographs showing the situation at 24 months' follow-up.

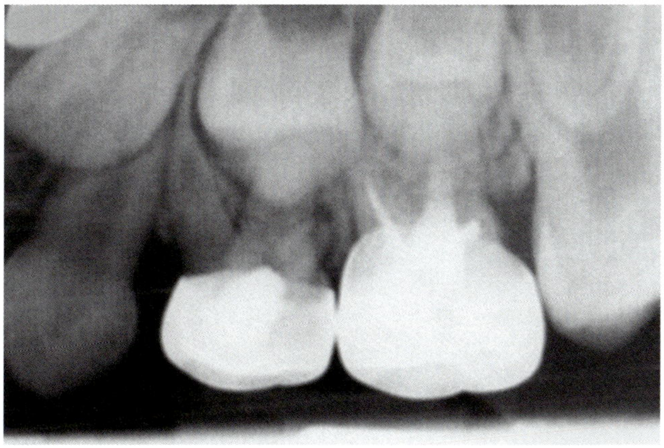

Fig. 16-6 Radiographs showing no evidence of any pathology in the pulp-treated teeth.

REFERENCES

1. Duggal MS, Nooh A, High AS. Response of the primary pulp to inflammation: a review of the Leeds studies and challenges for the future. Eur J Paediatr Dent 2002;2:111–114.
2. Huth KC, Paschos E, et al. Effectiveness of 4 pulpotomy techniques – randomised controlled trial. J Dent Res 2005;84:1144–1148.
3. Roberts JF, Attari N, Sherriff. The survival of resin modified glass ionomer and stainless steel crown restorations in primary molars, placed in a specialist paediatric dental practice. Br Dent J 2005;198:427–431.

ABBREVIATIONS

ALP	alkaline phosphatase
ALPL	liver/bone/kidney alkaline phosphatase
ASA	American Society of Anesthesiologists
ASA I	healthy patient, no medical problems
ASA II	patient with mild systemic disease
CNS	central nervous system
DD-I	dentin dysplasia type I
DD-II	dentin dysplasia type II
DD-III	dentin dysplasia type III
DI-I	dentinogenesis imperfecta type I
DI-II	dentinogenesis imperfecta type II
DI-III	dentinogenesis imperfecta type III
DSPP	dentin sialophosphoprotein
ECC	early childhood caries
ED	ectodermal dysplasia
FGF	fibroblast growth factor
GA	general anesthesia
GIC	glass-ionomer cement
GORD	gastroesophageal reflux disease
MIH	molar–incisor hypomineralization
MSX1	Msh homeobox 1
MTA	mineral trioxide aggregate
NC	nursing caries
NSAID	non-steroidal anti-inflammatory drug
PAX9	paired box gene 9
PDL	periodontal ligament
PMC	preformed metal crown
S-ECC	severe early childhood caries
SSC	stainless steel crown
TNAP	tissue–non-specific alkaline phosphatase
WHO	World Health Organization

INDEX